PERFECTLY CLEAR

THE PERFECT GUIDE TO CLEAR SKIN

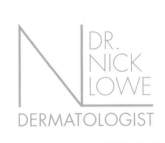

PERFECTLY CLEAR

THE PERFECT GUIDE TO CLEAR SKIN

BANISH ACNE, SPOTS AND BLEMISHES

Dr Nick Lowe MB, ChB, MD, FRCP
Consultant Dermatologist
Clinical Professor of Dermatology

Dr Philippa Lowe MB, ChB
Diploma in Dermatology
Skin Specialist Physician in Dermatology

Matador
9 Priory Business Park,
Wistow Road, Kibworth Beauchamp,
Leicestershire. LE8 0RX
Tel: 0116 279 2299
Email: books@troubador.co.uk
Web: www.troubador.co.uk/matador
Twitter: @matadorbooks

ISBN 978 1785890 833

British Library Cataloguing in Publication Data.
A catalogue record for this book is available from the British Library.

Typeset in 11pt Proxima Nova by Troubador Publishing Ltd, Leicester, UK

Matador is an imprint of Troubador Publishing Ltd

'There is no single disease, which causes more psychic trauma, more maladjustment between parents and children, more general insecurity and feelings of inferiority than does acne.'

Dr Marion Sulzberger, pioneer in dermatology

CONTENTS

INTRODUCTION

DO YOU HAVE ACNE, SPOTS, BLEMISHES? THIS BOOK WILL
HELP YOU

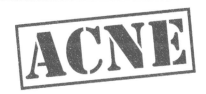

80% of us will have some acne at some time. With this book, you will be informed about how best to clear your spots, often by your own actions, with diet and lifestyle changes and with anti-blemish products you can buy or that can be prescribed by your doctor or dermatologist.

The reality is that many people with spots, oily skin and blackheads have tried many different treatments without much success or if they have improved their skin the problem just comes back. We will help you stop this 'acne cycle'.

This book will empower you with all the information and guidance you need to get the great clear skin you so want and deserve.

ACNE IS VERY COMMON

Acne is one of the leading causes of visits to doctors because of its frequency and its occurrence on the very visible skin of our faces.

MORE THAN 80% OF US WILL GET ACNE AT SOME TIME

Acne can affect any age group; most commonly it starts in adolescence, but many women have acne in their 20s, 30s or even 40s and 50s. In some women it continues throughout their adult life.

WHAT IS MEANT BY ACNE, SPOTS, BLEMISHES AND BREAKOUTS?

'Acne', 'spots', 'blemishes' and 'breakouts' are all terms for the same skin problem, a specific skin disease — acne, which is caused by hormones, with increased harmful bacteria leading to oily skin, blackheads, whiteheads and inflamed spots. The condition, which is sometimes associated with stress, certain medicines, acne-forming creams and cosmetics, or pregnancy, can be disfiguring, embarrassing and distressing.

THIS BOOK WILL HELP YOU GET CONTROL AND GET CLEAR SKIN.

CHAPTER 1

MILD OR SEVERE ACNE?

KNOWING WHICH HELPS YOU FIND THE BEST TREATMENT

GRADE 1: MILD ACNE

Mild acne may be a matter of just a few occasional red spots, blackheads, whiteheads and slight oiliness, usually on the face. With this type of acne you can help yourself: you can look for triggers (see chapter 4), change your diet (see chapter 5) and buy non-prescription products (see chapter 12).

> 66 Though it is classed as 'mild' by doctors, it can be anything but mild to you. 99

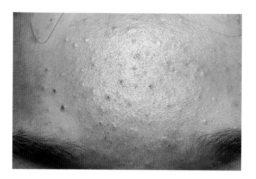

Grade 1 acne: mild early acne with skin oiliness and blackheads on the forehead

You can also get acne on the back.

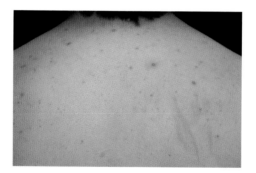

Grade 1 back acne: many small red inflamed acne spots on the back. This teenage girl with mild acne is a sportswoman and the friction from her tight sports tops aggravated her acne.

GRADE 2: MODERATE ACNE

This grade of acne has inflamed red spots usually on the forehead, nose, cheeks and chin. For many people, acne does not worsen beyond this annoying stage. You can buy our acclenz™ for this type of acne. (See chapters 4, 5 and 6 for lifestyle and diet changes will help.)

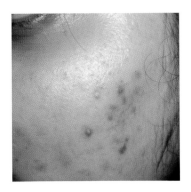

Grade 2 acne: red spots on the lower face in a young woman with moderate acne

GRADE 3: SEVERE ACNE

In severe acne inflamed spots are frequent, as well as blackheads, whiteheads and skin oiliness of the forehead and nose area. These require varied treatments, combining our acclenz™ products with prescription treatments (see chapters 7 and 8).

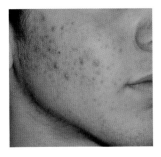

Grade 3 acne: whiteheads and inflamed spots in severe acne

GRADE 4: VERY SEVERE ACNE

If you have very severe acne you will have many red, painful spots and swollen skin. These may be very damaging to your confidence – really embarrassing and depressing. Again, the treatment is likely to be a combination of products available for you to buy and prescription-only treatments from a skin specialist physician (see chapters 7 and 8).

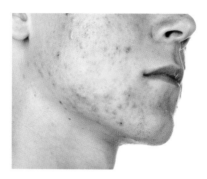

Grade 4 acne: many larger, red, inflamed, often painful bumps, plus early red raised scars, in very severe acne

GRADE 5: EXTREMELY SEVERE ACNE

When acne is as severe as this, you develop larger, painful, red lesions called nodules. These raised spots go deeper into the skin, are more intensely inflamed and are much more likely to leave scars (see chapters 8 and 9).

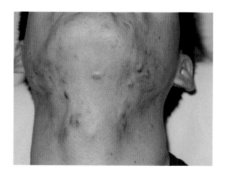

Grade 5 acne: severe nodules in extremely severe acne

GRADE 6: MOST SEVERE ACNE

In the most severe type of acne, in addition to nodules and large red bumps, burst nodules under the skin result in pus-filled sacs or cysts. These need to be treated using a combination of prescription gels and creams, plus oral medication (including antibiotics), hormone-blocking medicines and oral isotretinoin – known as Roaccutane in the UK and Accutane in the USA (see chapter 8).

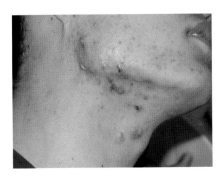

Grade 6 acne: most severe acne – will need prescription treatments – possibly Roaccutane.

A rare, but extremely severe, type of acne, which can cause fevers, chills and joint pains, is called acne fulminans.

This occurs as a result of severely inflamed acne releasing inflammatory chemicals into the body called cytokines, which produce fevers, chills, aches and joint pain – similar to a very bad case of flu.

Dermatologists treat acne fulminans with oral antibiotics, cortisone, anti- inflammation medicines and Roaccutane.

CHAPTER 2
WHY DO YOU GET ACNE?

KNOWLEDGE GIVES YOU THE POWER TO HELP YOUR SKIN

THE BOTTOM LINE IS THAT HORMONES CAUSE ACNE

Hormones produced during teenage years are called androgens. Androgens are responsible in both boys and girls for changes of voice and hair growth, and in boys the start of beards. Skin becomes oily as a result of androgens. The combination of androgens and oestrogens in girls is responsible for their normal maturation and sexual development.

Unfortunately, androgens also start the chain of events that result in acne. Androgens, male hormones, occur in both women and men and cause acne.

ANDROGENS START ACNE

Why does acne start and get worse?

Your body makes more androgen hormones as teenagers, under stress, before menstruation, with some dairy products, some medicines and contraceptives, and during and after pregnancy.

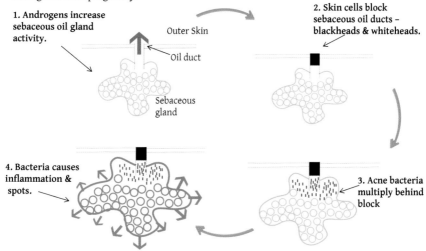

1. Androgens increase sebaceous oil gland activity.

Outer Skin

Oil duct

Sebaceous gland

2. Skin cells block sebaceous oil ducts – blackheads & whiteheads.

4. Bacteria causes inflammation & spots.

3. Acne bacteria multiply behind block

SEE IF THE FOLLOWING QUESTIONS GIVE YOU A CLUE AS TO WHY YOU HAVE MORE CHANCE OF GETTING ACNE.

Was there any acne in your family?

In some families the sebaceous oil glands tend to have greater sensitivity to the hormones that cause acne.

What about your diet?

Some foods and drinks trigger acne or make it worse (see chapter 5).

Are you living with a high level of stress?

Stress can cause acne and by coping with stress you may be able to improve your acne. We will help you de-stress (see chapter 6).

Do you sleep badly?

Poor sleep and inadequate rest create stress, and in doing so may make acne worse (see chapter 6).

Could your cosmetics be causing acne?

Some cosmetics and creams can make acne-prone skin worse; we call these **comedogenic** products (from **comedone**, the medical term for blackhead) (see chapter 4).

Could you be using medication that causes acne?

Some medicines can cause acne. We will guide you so that you can avoid them wherever possible and ask your doctor about them (see chapter 4).

SOME OTHER THINGS TO CONSIDER

Pregnancy can help improve acne in some, but can make it worse in others.

We will discuss acne in pregnancy and tell you which treatments are safe during pregnancy and which you must avoid (see chapter 9).

Acne seems to be worse in some people in the summer.

Find out why this may be and what to do (see chapter 4).

Even some clothes can make acne worse.

This is mainly to do with sweating and friction. Comedones result from occlusion (blockage) of the pores of the skin (see chapter 4).

When does acne usually start?

Most commonly it begins during the teenage or even pre-teenage years, when androgen hormone levels rise.

Often the first signs are increased skin oiliness in forehead, nose, cheeks and chin, together with blackheads and whiteheads. It can also start in adult life – we will discuss the reason for this later in the chapter.

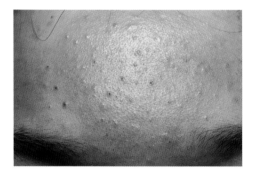

Early acne in a teenager with oily skin, and blackheads and whiteheads on the forehead – the earliest signs of acne

Infants with acne

Acne occurs in infants quite frequently and is known as infantile acne. We reassure mothers of children with infantile acne that it rarely requires treatment and will clear of its own accord.

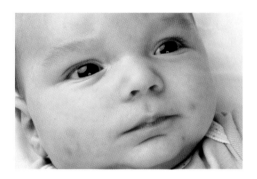

Infant with acne – a lovely baby boy with some acne spots on his cheeks. These will clear without treatment.

Why do we need sebaceous glands?

During human evolution our prehistoric ancestors had a considerable covering of hair to protect their bodies. To make hair waterproof, weatherproof and more resistant to all sorts of environmental assaults, the sebaceous glands produced oil to coat the hair. This oil does not help moisturize your skin but it does help with skin healing. Sebaceous glands are most frequent in the central face, forehead, nose, and chin, front chest, upper back and shoulders, that is, acne areas.

A blockage of the sebaceous duct becomes a blackhead when it is exposed to air because oxidation causes it to darken. A blockage that is not open to the air remains white and is called a whitehead.

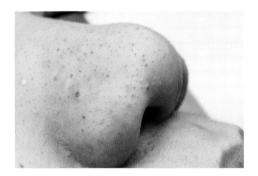

Why blackheads? Sebaceous duct plugs turn black on exposure to air.

Blockage of the sebaceous ducts and increased oil secretion behind the blackhead or whitehead allow the acne bacteria (proprionibacterium acnes or p. acnes) to multiply in the low-oxygen, warm, oily environment. The skin then tries to kill and control these bacteria by sending inflammation cells to the area to kill the bacteria. Unfortunately, these cells also lead to red acne spots.

After adolescence, sebaceous oil glands usually become more resistant to androgens and stop reacting to them. Your acne may clear or improve at this stage.

Why do some of us continue to get acne?

Unfortunately some people produce too much androgen and that continues to trigger the acne. In some women this is a result of a condition called polycystic ovarian syndrome (PCOS) (see chapter 8).

Some men are over-reactive to normal levels of androgens and continue to produce excessive sebaceous oil, causing blackheads and increased p. acnes bacteria.

HOW ACNE EVOLVES

Formation of Skin Pimples and Acne

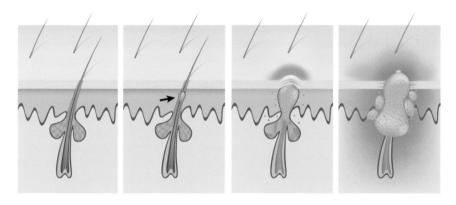

1. Healthy follicle

2. Duct clogged by dead cells, sebum starts to accumulate

3. Bacterial infection, inflammation triggered, - - pimple

4. Follicle ruptures, pustule with fluid formed - acne

CHAPTER 3

ACNE IMITATORS

RED SPOTS THAT ARE NOT ACNE

OTHER CONDITIONS THAT LOOK LIKE ACNE

ROSACEA (ROSE-AY-SHA)

One of the most common acne imitators is a skin disease called rosacea, which used to be called adult acne. It is a different disease, with skin redness and red pimples but without blackheads and whiteheads.

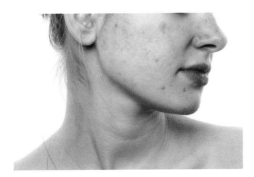

Rosacea: an acne imitator. This woman has red spots and redness on her nose and cheeks, together with 'thread veins'.

Some people with acne develop rosacea as well and have both conditions at the same time. Rosacea may begin as a tendency to flush or blush easily. If the disease worsens, enlarged blood vessels (telangiectasia) and pimples begin to appear.

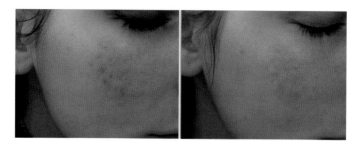

Rosacea: classical red, acne-like, pimples under the skin before and after treatment. It is often confused with acne.

ROSACEA TREATMENTS AT OUR CLINIC

Rosacea can be treated; we prescribe a combination of antibiotic pills and skin creams such as metronidazole, azelaic acid or ivermectin.

A few sessions of intense-pulsed-light treatment or blood-vessel-targeted lasers reduce face redness further.

Occasionally, for more severe rosacea we prescribe Roaccutane.

OTHER ACNE IMITATORS

PERIORAL DERMATITIS

Spots and redness around the mouth and chin are sometimes a result of perioral dermatitis, a condition that is more common in women. It can be caused by prescription or non-prescription cortisone creams e.g. hydrocortisone cream. It's a good rule to avoid putting cortisone creams on your face, unless prescribed by a skin specialist or dermatologist for a few rare skin conditions. Perioral dermatitis is treated in the same way as rosacea – see above.

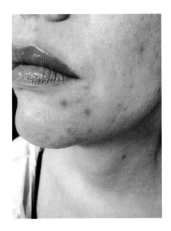

Perioral dermatitis

CHAPTER 4

WHAT CAN MAKE ACNE WORSE?

IDENTIFY AND REMOVE YOUR ACNE TRIGGERS

There are many things that can trigger or worsen acne.

CONTRACEPTIVE PILLS AND ACNE

Oral contraceptives usually contain the hormones oestrogen and progesterone, which can increase the effects of androgens on the sebaceous glands.

The oral contraceptives that tend to improve acne usually contain higher oestrogen levels and other ingredients that block androgen action, but they carry a higher risk of deep vein thrombosis (blood clots in the leg veins), strokes and a variety of other serious problems, including migraines and raised blood pressure. These side effects are more likely to occur if you are also a smoker – another reason to quit smoking if you are taking an oral contraceptive.

So whether taking oral contraceptives will worsen or help your acne is likely to depend on the type you use. This is something for you to discuss with your GP, gynaecologist, skin specialist doctor or dermatologist.

POLYCYSTIC OVARIAN SYNDROME (PCOS) AND PERSISTING ACNE

Women with a condition called polycystic ovarian syndrome (PCOS) have either increased levels of androgen or an increased sebaceous gland reaction to normal androgen levels.

PCOS patients can be helped by some oral contraceptives and other medicines (e.g. spironolactone) that block androgens (see chapter 8).

PREGNANCY CAN CLEAR OR WORSEN ACNE

Women who have acne usually find it improves when they become pregnant. The acne may or may not come back after pregnancy (see chapter 9).

There are however some woman who will continue to get worse during pregnancy. The reasons for this are to do with changing hormone levels.

STRESS MAKES ACNE WORSE

Most of us know that stress can indeed worsen acne. Several well-conducted research studies have proved this. One, for example, showed that university students with stress from end-of-term exams get more acne.

The body copes with stress by releasing the hormone cortisone, one side effect of which is to cause acne by an androgen-like effect on the skin and sebaceous glands (see chapter 6).

WHAT MEDICINES CAN CAUSE ACNE?

Some patients treated with cortisones for diseases such as rheumatoid arthritis can develop cortisone-related acne.

Other medicines that can induce acne include certain antidepressants, including lithium, (which is prescribed for bipolar disorders and severe depression), and some anti-epileptic medicines, one of the most common being phenobarbitone.

Give your doctor a full medicine history to enable him or her to pinpoint any possible links between your acne and medicines you have been taking; the doctor will often be able to prescribe an alternative.

THINGS THAT MAY MAKE ACNE WORSE

Androgens, e.g. body-building hormones
Diet – chapter 5
Pregnancy – chapter 9
Stress – chapter 6
Medications
Skincare products and make-up

COMEDOGENIC SKINCARE PRODUCTS AND COSMETICS

Some skincare and cosmetic products – e.g. heavy moisturizers and make-up and some sunscreens – are described as comedogenic because they have a tendency to cause acne by blocking the opening of the oil glands.

Avoid buying skincare products and cosmetics containing comedogenic ingredients.

COMEDOGENIC INGREDIENTS

Algae extracts
Cetearyl alcohol
Coal tars
Cocoa butter
Coconut oil
Glyceryl stearate
Isopropyl isostearate
Isopropyl myristate
Isopropyl palmitate
Lanolin (acetylated)
Laureth 4
Laureth acid
Mink oil
Oleic acid
Oleth 3
Red algae
Sesame oil
Sodium lauryl sulphate
Soybean oil
Stearic acid

Creams and cosmetics labelled as **non-comedogenic** are less likely to cause acne.

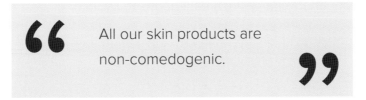

" All our skin products are non-comedogenic. "

CHAPTER 5

GOOD AND BAD FOODS AND ACNE

THOSE THAT HELP, THOSE THAT MAKE IT WORSE

Diet has a role in acne, though it is rarely food alone that causes acne. Keeping a diary, (recording foods eaten and the severity of your skin problem), may help you identify trigger foods.

A study published in the prestigious *Journal of the American Academy of Dermatology* in 2012, showed that people with moderate and severe acne were likely to consume large quantities of dairy products, sweets and milk chocolate.

There is more and more research to suggest that some diets are linked with acne. Processed refined carbohydrates (sugar, chocolate, sweets, white flour and white pasta) are the foods to avoid or at least go easy on. If you reduce these to 10% of your diet, you will decrease the action of the hormones that make skin oily, and, in turn, reduce acne.

In societies where little or no processed food is eaten, acne seems pretty rare.

CARBS – BAD AND GOOD

THE GLYCAEMIC INDEX (GI)

Carbohydrates can be divided into simple 'fast-acting' carbohydrates and complex or 'slow-release' carbohydrates. Foods are sometimes described as high or low glycaemic foods according to their effect on blood glucose levels, and different foods can be ranked on the Glycaemic Index (GI), the higher the GI the faster the rise in the blood glucose level. Pure glucose has a GI of 100.

GI range	Examples	
Low GI GOOD	55 or less	beans, lentils, soy, almonds, peanuts, walnuts, chickpeas, seeds (sunflower, flax, pumpkin, poppy, sesame), most whole intact grains, durum/spelt, wheat, oats, rye, rice, barley, most vegetables, most fruits, (peaches, strawberries, mangoes), mushrooms, chillies
Medium GI	56–69	whole wheat, pitta bread, basmati rice, unpeeled boiled potatoes, grape juice, raisins, prunes, cranberry juice, ice cream, sucrose, bananas
High GI BAD	70 and above	white flour, bread, white rice, corn flakes, most breakfast cereals, glucose, potato crisps, pretzels, bagels

Bad or simple carbohydrates, e.g. glucose and sugar, which are ranked high on the glycaemic index, release energy quickly into the body, making blood glucose levels soar. Foods containing 'bad carbs' include things like sweets, syrup, white bread, white pasta and desserts. They give short-lived energy but leave us feeling tired afterwards. They are linked to obesity and insulin-resistance, and increase the risk of diabetes and premature ageing.

These foods seem to make acne worse, by increasing skin response to androgens.

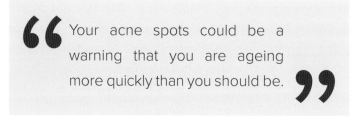

> Your acne spots could be a warning that you are ageing more quickly than you should be.

GOOD OR COMPLEX CARBOHYDRATES

Good or complex carbohydrates, e.g. whole wheat, those that rank low on the glycaemic index, release their energy more slowly, are better for your health and your skin, and are therefore less likely to aggravate acne (see table 'The glycaemic index rating of some foods').

PROTEINS ARE GOOD

Proteins provide us with amino acids, which are essential for building cells, including those in the skin, hair and nails. Proteins also play a vital part in the production of collagen and elastin — necessary for youthful-looking skin with a good texture and tone.

Good sources of protein include lean meat, fish, nuts, tofu, soya, eggs, cheese, beans and lentils.

BETTER-FOR-YOU FATS

'Good' fats are an important source of energy and also play a role in skin health. They help the skin produce its own natural fats, or lipids, which act as a barrier against water loss and keep skin feeling smooth and supple. They help reduce inflamed skin in acne.

SOME 'BETTER-FOR-YOU-FATS'

Monounsaturates

Monounsaturates are found in olive oil, avocados, seeds and nuts.

Polyunsaturates

Polyunsaturates are found in most vegetable oils, including corn, rapeseed and sunflower, and also oily fish.

DAIRY PRODUCTS MAKE ACNE WORSE

Dairy products can worsen acne because dairy cattle are fed hormones to increase milk production. If traces of these hormones are present in dairy foods they can cause or aggravate acne.

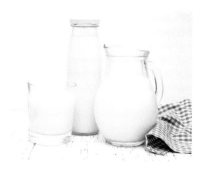

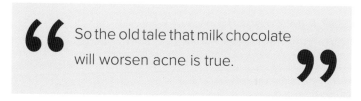

" So the old tale that milk chocolate will worsen acne is true. "

Skimmed milk is **particularly** bad for your acne.

The association between milk intake and teenage acne was greatest with skimmed (non-fat milk). Studies showed that when the skimmed milk was analysed there was a high GI compared to whole milk, which may worsen acne.

HOW TO REDUCE YOUR DAIRY INTAKE

Try soya milk and other milk substitutes – if you really *love* milk, drink small amounts of whole fat milk instead of skimmed milk, and eat dark chocolate instead of milk chocolate.

WHAT TO EAT FOR CLEAR SKIN

What you eat can be just as important as the creams you put on your skin. If you want radiant and healthy skin, here are some nutrient ingredients to consider.

1. VITAMIN A

Vitamin A plays an important role in skin cell formation, and getting adequate (but not excessive) amounts is beneficial for people with acne. Some acne creams and medicines are developed from vitamin A.

Foods containing vitamin A
Beta carotene, which is converted to vitamin A in the body, is found in orange-coloured foods, such as carrots, sweet potato, pumpkin, mangoes and butternut squash. It's safer to get vitamin A from foods rather than supplements. Too much vitamin A supplement is toxic to the body and can result in dangerous side effects, including foetal defects in pregnant women.

2. VITAMIN E

Vitamin E is a powerful antioxidant that helps to prevent premature ageing and promotes smooth, supple skin. The body can't produce vitamin E, so it gets it from the foods you eat. Vitamin E helps vitamin A to work on your skin, thereby helping acne.

Foods containing vitamin E
Vitamin E is found in many nuts, fruits and vegetables, and in olive oil, sunflower oil and wheat-germ oil.

3. LYCOPENE

Lycopene gives tomatoes their red colour and is an excellent antioxidant, helping to prevent the skin from being damaged by free radicals caused by inflammation e.g. acne and UV rays.

Foods containing lycopene
Tinned tomatoes contain even more lycopene than fresh – so get your daily dose with homemade pasta sauces and soups.

TOMATOES

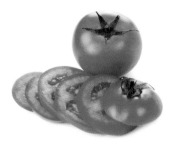

Cooked and canned tomatoes have three times the amount of lycopene you would get from a fresh uncooked tomato.

4. OMEGA 3 FATTY ACIDS

Omega 3 and 6 fatty acids from oily fish help skin to be healthier and less inflamed.

You need to eat two portions of oily fish every week for maximum benefit. Fish oil supplements can be a good option.

Foods containing omega 3 fatty acids

The richest sources of omega fatty acids are fish such as sardines, mackerel, tuna and salmon. Alternatives include flax seeds and oil, hemp seeds and oil, walnuts, soybeans, and pumpkin seeds and oil.

SALMON AND OILY FISH

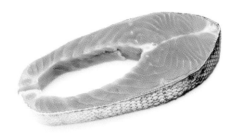

Herrings, mackerel, sardines, salmon and tuna keep skin moisturized, healthy and less inflamed.

5. SELENIUM

As we get older skin loses some of its natural elasticity and becomes more prone to wrinkles. Inflamed acne can damage collagen and elastin.

Selenium is an antioxidant mineral that helps to protect the skin from inflammation and sun damage and preserves elastin, a protein that keeps the skin smooth and tight.

Foods containing selenium

Sources of selenium include Brazil nuts, fresh and saltwater fish, beef, poultry, wheat germ and brown rice. It's best to get selenium from food rather than supplements. Too much selenium supplement can be toxic.

6. ZINC

Zinc speeds up skin renewal, protects cell membranes and controls sebaceous oil gland activity — a very important cause of acne.

Foods containing zinc
Sources of zinc include lentils, black-eyed peas, soybeans, oysters, lobster, lean beef, crab, wheat germ, skinless chicken and turkey, lean lamb, clams, mussels, pumpkin seeds, yogurt, cashews, peanuts and sunflower seeds.

7. VITAMIN B3 (NIACIN/NIACINAMIDE)

Vitamin B3 helps acne by reducing skin inflammation and improving the skin's ability to be a protective barrier.

Foods containing vitamin B3
Sources of vitamin B3 include oily fish (especially tuna), chicken, turkey, mushrooms, kale, broccoli, peanuts, beans and cereal.

KALE

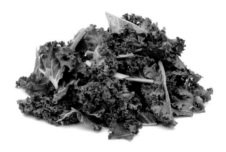

Kale is a great source of niacin/niacinamide, which is essential for good, clear skin.

8. MONOUNSATURATED FATTY ACIDS

Monounsaturated fats don't just protect heart health, lower cholesterol and help fight inflammation from acne. They also contain iron and copper, which defend against free radicals and are involved in collagen production, promoting skin elasticity.

Foods containing monosaturated fatty acids
Monosaturated fatty acids are found in foods like avocados, seeds and nuts. Too many people watching their weight cut avocado from their diet. One avocado provides 320 calories and 29g of fat, but the fats are monounsaturated and help lower total cholesterol, making them a healthy choice.

AVOCADO

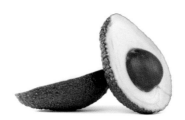

These 'salad' fruits are rich in the potassium, vitamins and fats we all need. they also contain Vitamin E, which helps skin heal and regenerate.

9. DARK CHOCOLATE

We love dark chocolate! Dark chocolate doesn't just taste good, it also contains antioxidants, which can reduce the skin damage caused by acne inflammation. But being dairy-free it doesn't also aggravate acne as milk chocolate does.

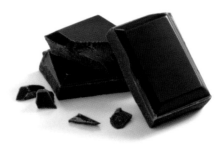

Dark chocolate contains cocoa and is a healthy pleasure you can enjoy. Dark chocolate is high in antioxidants, which aid the heart and skin, reducing acne inflammation.

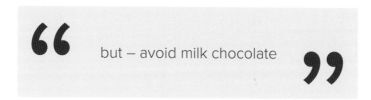

" but – avoid milk chocolate "

10. VITAMIN C

Vitamin C, the natural antioxidant, is needed for healthy blood vessels, collagen and joint health, and for reducing inflamed acne. It may help reduce scar severity after acne by helping to make new collagen in your skin.

Foods containing vitamin C
Citrus fruits, such as oranges and lemons, and fresh citrus fruit juices are a great source of vitamin C, as are some of the so-called super fruits, such as goji, acai, blueberries and raspberries, also green salads and green vegetables.

BLUEBERRIES

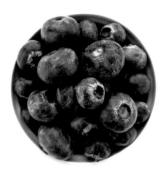

Blueberries contain antioxidant protectants called flavonoids, which help to reduce sugar damage (glycation) to skin cells.

RASPBERRIES

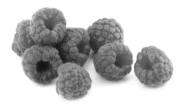

Raspberries contain powerful skin protectants called rutinosides, which reduce sun damage and inflammation to the skin.

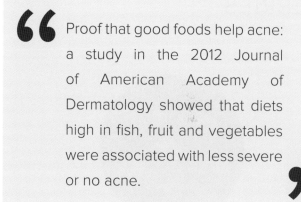
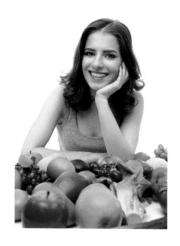

Eat plenty of different coloured fruits and vegetables for a good mix of antioxidants and nutrients that will help protect your skin from damage, help skin repair itself and reduce inflammation from your acne.

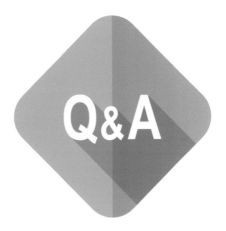

QUESTIONS AND ANSWERS ABOUT FOOD AND DRINK

Q: Are tea and coffee bad for the skin?

A: (Nick) They aren't bad for the skin per se, but if you have too many cups a day, you may feel shaky and stressed from too much caffeine. Coffee is a good source for niacinamide, which helps acne. One or two cups supply enough niacinamide for a day.

If you drink green tea, you'll be getting extra antioxidants. If you flush easily or suffer from rosacea, very hot tea and coffee may make your face redder. Let them cool.

Q: Should I give up chocolate for the sake of my skin?

A: (Philippa) If you are acne-prone, but love your chocolate, go for dark rather than milk chocolate. Milk chocolate may contain traces of acne-causing hormones. It's fine to nibble on a little dark chocolate. Chocolate with a high cocoa content contains antioxidants such as procyanidin, which can help all kinds of health problems and may help to reduce inflamed acne.

Q: Does eating too much sugar, desserts or sweets give me spots?

A: (Philippa) Yes, any of these foods that have high glycaemic content may worsen your acne. One possible way they do this is by increasing the 'acne-forming' action of your hormones. Look for low glycaemic treats instead.

Q: Can vitamin supplements help my acne?

A: (Philippa) There's no substitute for a healthy balanced diet, but we do recommend omega 3 supplements to boost skin health and improve acne. Omega 3 oils come from oily fish (salmon, herring, and mackerel), which we often don't eat enough of. They fight inflammation and promote healing. Niacinamide and zinc have also been shown to be beneficial for acne. Moderate doses of vitamin A supplement, 5000 units per day, may help acne.

CHAPTER 6

STRESS MAKES ACNE WORSE

HOW THE WAY YOU FEEL AFFECTS THE WAY YOU LOOK –
HOW TO DE-STRESS YOURSELF TO HELP YOUR SKIN

Irritable? Anxious? Trouble sleeping? You could be stressed. Some stress in your life is fine. It gets you up in the morning! In fact, some people positively thrive on it. But when you feel uptight, cranky or panicky on a regular basis it shows in your face with more spots, and it is time to reduce that stress.

WHAT ARE YOUR STRESS TRIGGERS?

Figuring out what is winding you up helps you to put it in perspective. Sometimes it's just day-to-day stuff that needles away at you. At other times, it is life's big moments.

Common stressors include

School and university exams
Getting married
Getting divorced or ending a relationship

Moving home
Starting a new job/losing your job
Bereavement

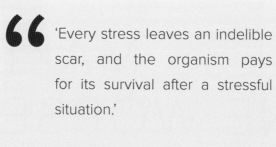

'Every stress leaves an indelible scar, and the organism pays for its survival after a stressful situation.'

Hans Selye, endocrinologist who first coined the word 'stress'

HOW STRESS MESSES WITH MORE THAN YOUR HEAD

Stress sets off a chain reaction in the body. It causes extra hormones, including cortisol, to be released by your adrenal glands. This is the body's natural defence system in a crisis and known as the fight or flight response – to help us respond when confronted by danger.

These hormone surges stimulate your sebaceous glands to produce more oil and more acne.

We frequently see people in our clinics who say that their breakouts get worse during a period of stress. This ties in with research done in the USA showing that women university students always had more breakouts before their end-of-year exams.

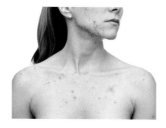

Female university students were shown to get more acne when stressed by end of year examinations.

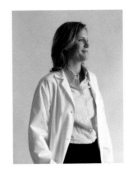

Philippa's bright idea! My de-stress tip:

" At times when I feel under pressure, I've found it helpful to do a 'stress audit'. I make two lists, one with all the negative stuff and the other with all the things that make me feel happy and chilled, such as my kids, my husband, running outdoors and catching up with my girlfriends. As well as trying to work out ways of dealing with the stress-causers, I find it useful to think about the positives when I feel tense to help me regain a sense of balance. "

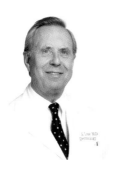

Nick's way of coping with stress:

" I have recently discovered the 'mindfulness' method of grounding myself and reducing stress. This is an excellent programme recently developed by psychiatrists at Oxford University. A valuable resource is the book and CD set *Mindfulness: A practical guide to finding peace in a frantic world* by Mark Williams and Danny Penman, published by Piatkus. "

STRESS-BEATING STRATEGIES

GET MOVING

Exercise is good for your health – it releases endorphins – feel-good hormones – keeping stress at bay. It lowers your blood pressure, protects against brittle bones and burns calories. Schedule exercise into your day as a regular appointment.

Do something you like, whether that's yoga, pilates, dance classes, swimming, walking or playing a sport – that way you'll be sure to keep it up.

LEARN TO SAY NO

If you feel put upon, say so. You can't please all the people all the time.

PRIORITIZE

Don't sweat over what won't bother you in a few months' or a year's time.

KEEP RHYTHM IN YOUR LIFE

The body (and skin) responds well to a routine, such as going to bed and waking up at the same time each day and sticking to regular meal times, rather than skipping meals.

TRY MEDITATING

One of our favourites is listening to a mindfulness CD, but you can find your own preferred method.

Try repeating the same word over and over slowly in your mind for ten to fifteen minutes.

If you take a meditation class, you'll be given a word or 'mantra' to say, but you can just as easily choose your own.

Alternatively, visualize being in your favourite place, such as by the sea, climbing a mountain or working in your garden. Close your eyes and take yourself there for a few minutes, slowing your breathing.

UNWIND WITH A MUSCLE-RELAXATION TECHNIQUE

Find a quiet place where you won't be disturbed.

Lie flat or sit in a chair.

Tense, then relax your muscle groups starting with your feet and working all the way up your body to the neck area.

Or try this simple breathing exercise:

b r e a t h e … slowly and calmly. Conscious deep breathing calms. Breathe out through your mouth, pulling your abdomen in for a count of five. Hold for five, and then inhale for five counts, letting your abdomen expand as you are breathing in. Repeat five times.

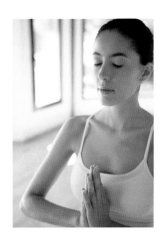

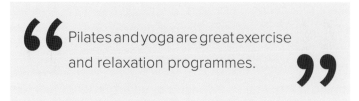

> **Pilates and yoga are great exercise and relaxation programmes.**

AND HERE'S HOW <u>NOT</u> TO SOOTHE STRESS...

SMOKING

Cigarettes, with their nicotine content, actually make your body more stressed and exacerbate your stress acne.

It's not easy to quit: it takes great willpower, though nicotine release patches and electronic cigarettes may help. Hypnotherapy can also help people to quit.

Alcohol can worsen face redness and inflamed acne

Too much alcohol causes stress. Rather than using alcohol as a prop, address the problems. If you have a real problem find an Alcoholics Anonymous group in your area.

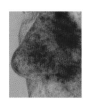

Alcohol increases blood flow to the face and nose – this makes rosacea and inflamed acne worse.

> **Better sleep helps de-stress.**

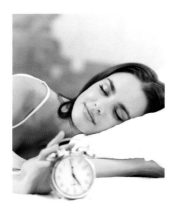

Winding down for up to an hour before going to bed really helps. A warm bath is not only de-stressing, but will start to stimulate melatonin, 'sleep hormone', production.

Cut down or avoid tea, coffee and other caffeinated drinks from mid-afternoon onwards as their stimulating effects remain in your system for hours. Alcohol disturbs sleep too.

CHAPTER 7

DIY TREATMENTS FOR ACNE

EMPOWER YOURSELF TO GET CLEAR SKIN

Acne is caused by hormones but there are multiple triggers that can make it worse. Combining treatments targets these several acne triggers, but also different skin types need different treatments. You may not tolerate some treatments but do really well with others.

EFFECTIVE TREATMENTS ALSO REDUCE RISK OF SCARRING

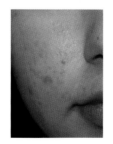 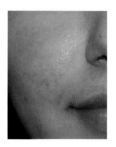

Non-prescription cream products help mild acne.

How can you make your acne better and get clear skin?

Many people with acne will try self-treatment before seeing a physician.

5% of acne patients wait over a year before seeing a GP, a skin specialist physician or a dermatologist.

25% of people with acne will never seek a consultation with a physician or skin specialist and will use non-prescription products or give up on treatment altogether.

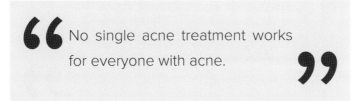

> No single acne treatment works for everyone with acne.

IDENTIFY YOUR SKIN TYPE TO HELP CHOOSE THE BEST TREATMENT COMBINATIONS

Skin type	Recommended treatment
Normal skin with acne	Normal cleanser Most anti-acne products
Sensitive skin with acne	Gentle cleansers Gentle anti-acne products
Dry skin with acne	Moisture cleanser Gentle anti-acne products
Oily skin with acne	Oil-reducing creams Most anti-acne products
Combination oily/dry skin with acne	Oil-reducing creams Moisturisers to dry areas Most anti-acne products

RECOMMENDED TREATMENTS FOR DIFFERENT SKIN TYPES

These different skin types need different treatment approaches. You can use non-prescription products in combination with prescription treatments. We will help you to get the right combination for your skin type because many creams, gels and lotions can be too drying or irritating for sensitive, dry and even apparently normal skin. Our acclenz™ products can be used for acne on all skin types including sensitive and dry skin.

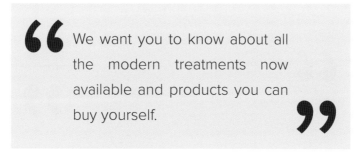

> **"** We want you to know about all the modern treatments now available and products you can buy yourself. **"**

WHAT CAN YOU DO TO HELP YOURSELF?

There is a wide range of over-the-counter or non-prescription products available for treating your acne.

TYPES OF NON-PRESCRIPTION PRODUCTS FOR ACNE

Acne cleansers
Anti-blemish creams, lotions, gels and masks
Exfoliation and skin-peeling treatments
Spot gels
Vitamins and supplements

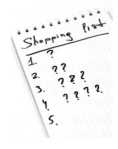

WHAT SHOULD I LOOK FOR IN ANTI-ACNE PRODUCTS?

The ingredients that are available in many non-prescription anti-acne products include the following:

Salicylic acid

Salicylic acid can be obtained from natural sources – it is often derived from witch hazel – or it can be manufactured.

It is a beta-hydroxy acid that helps to shed outer skin layers or epidermis and a **comedolytic**, that is, it reduces blackhead and whitehead formation. It can also enhance the action of other topical anti-acne ingredients.

In some products it can irritate the skin.

Benzoyl peroxide

Benzoyl peroxide (BPO) comes in a low strength – usually 2.5% – in some non-prescription creams, gels, lotions and washes.

It kills acne bacteria and is often combined with topical antibiotics.

It is helpful for some patients but you may find it too drying and it can irritate the skin. It is usually recommended that people use it at night to avoid too much skin irritancy. It also bleaches dark clothes.

Retinoids

Retinol, retinaldehyde, retinyl palmitate – these are all strengths of Vitamin-A- related ingredients called retinoids. Nonprescription retinoids can help mild acne but are not as effective as prescription retinoids.

Sulphur

Sulphur is a long-used ingredient in non-prescription products for acne. It has an effect against the redness or inflammation of acne and may help to absorb skin surface oils produced by sebaceous glands.

It has modest benefits for acne and can be combined with salicylic acid. It can be applied to local spots or larger skin areas. Sulphur is available in creams, masks and peels.

It may be drying for your skin, in which case reduce the frequency of application to two or three nights per week.

Some products containing sulphur smell of bad eggs!

Eucalyptus oil

Eucalyptus oil, which is available as a natural extract, has antiseptic properties. Apply to local red spots twice daily with a cotton bud. It does not reduce blackheads or reduce sebaceous oils and so needs to be used with other products containing anti-blackhead and anti-sebaceous ingredients. We will discuss these later.

OUR NEW ACCLENZ™ RANGE OF PRODUCTS YOU CAN BUY ONLINE OR FROM SELECTED SHOPS WITHOUT PRESCRIPTION

WHY DID WE DEVELOP THESE PRODUCTS?

There are relatively few anti-acne ingredients in existing products and some of these other products can be irritating or too drying for many people, especially if they have sensitive skin.

We targeted the reasons you get blemishes and spots, from hormones to sebaceous oil, from bacteria causing inflammation to medicines, from creams to cosmetics.

Looking at these acne 'triggers' that lead to acne, we selected active ingredients and combined them as the acclenz™ complex of products. Testing showed that these improve blemishes quickly, maintain skin quality after improvement and are well tolerated by all skin types, including sensitive skin.

Laboratory testing at an internationally respected UK centre proved acclenz™ products killed all acne bacteria, including those resistant to anti-acne antibiotics.

We have been able to achieve *synergistic* anti-acne benefit, that is, the total beneficial effects of the ingredients is greater in this combination than when are used separately. At the same time, we have reduced the unwanted effects of many products – skin irritancy, dryness and redness problems. The active ingredients are at low concentration and can be made available without a prescription.

> " Our new products contain the combination complex that we developed called acclenz™ "

ACCLENZ™ INGREDIENTS

a	Antioxidants	vitamins A, C and E, and goji extracts
c	Calming agents	chamomile, allantoin, niacinamide
cl	Clearing agents	salicylic acid, witch hazel, niacinamide
e	Eucalyptus extract	kills acne bacteria
n	Niacinamide	reduces inflammation, discolouration and acne damage
z	Zinc PCA	reduces oil and repairs skin barrier

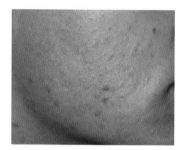 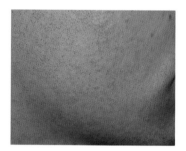

Before and after non-prescription acclenz™ products for mild acne

WHAT ARE OUR ACCLENZ™ INGREDIENTS AND WHAT DO THEY DO?

Antioxidants

Antioxidants reduce the damage to your skin caused by the bacteria responsible for inflammation and painful spots. The antioxidants used in acclenz™ are vitamins A, C and E, and goji and acai extracts.

Skin-calming agents

Skin-calming agents include natural and synthetic salicylic acids, chamomile, niacinamide and allantoin, all of which reduce the redness and inflammation. They also help your skin tolerate topical prescription medicines such as retinoids (see chapter 8).

Clear-skin agents

Microspheres of salicylic acid (minute particles specially formulated to release the active ingredient slowly) clear lesions without causing skin irritation.

Chlorhexidine

Chlorhexidine is an antibacterial, antiseptic, ingredient that targets acne bacteria. We use it in very dilute quantities, below levels that can irritate.

Eucalyptus extract

Eucalyptus extract is known to reduce bacteria numbers and skin redness. It has antiseptic and anti-inflammatory properties.

Niacinamide

Niacinamide – a form of vitamin B3 – is beneficial in numerous ways for acne: it has skin-calming activity, it reduces the production of sebaceous oil and it reduces darkened scars.

Zinc PCA

Zinc in the form of zinc PCA is similar to the skin's natural moisturizer. It reduces the oiliness of the skin and helps the anti-acne activity of niacinamide.

Together, niacinamide and zinc PCA also help to repair the damage to the skin barrier that acne spots cause.

OUR PATENT PENDING PRODUCTS FOR ACNE, FORMULATED WITH OUR ACCLENZ™ COMPLEX

Deep Action Blemish Serum
Apply to all the areas where you have spots after cleansing your skin morning and night.

Purify and Renew Foaming Cleanser
Use morning and night.

Oil Control Day Cream
If you have areas of oily skin on your face, apply to the oily skin twice daily.

Deep Down Clearing Mask
Apply weekly to the whole face.

Pore Refining Facial Polish
Use twice a week to cleanse and smooth.

Advanced Action Spot Gel
Dab onto any new and red spots up to four times a day, through make-up if necessary.

THE BENEFICIAL ACTIONS OF THESE ACCLENZ™ PRODUCTS

Proven blemish reduction
Reduced skin irritation
Blackhead removal
Killing of acne bacteria

Reduction of sebaceous oil on the skin surface
Maintain long-term clearance of spots
Improvement of dark scars or marks

ALL OUR PRODUCTS HAVE BEEN TESTED TO SHOW THEY ARE NON-IRRITATING AND SUITABLE FOR ALL SKIN TYPES INCLUDING SENSITIVE SKIN.

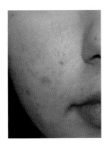 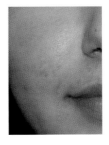

Before and after acclenz™ non-prescription products.

SELF-HELP SUMMARY FOR ACNE

HELP YOURSELF TO IMPROVE YOUR SKIN.

Treat your skin gently.
Cleanse it twice a day with a mild, oil-reducing cleanser. Try to resist scrubbing with washcloths and using exfoliating products too often, as this will only make your skin look angrier.

Don't use harsh toners and cleansers.
Toners and cleansers that smell very strongly of alcohol or with other ingredients that make your eyes water will be too drying and may damage your skin barrier.

Use a cleanser that moisturizes.
A cleanser that moisturizes will help your skin to be less dry when you use some prescription and non-prescription creams and gels and help you persist with these treatments. This is particularly important if you are prone to dry and sensitive skin. Aveeno, Cetaphil Lotion, Dermol 500 Lotion and Simple Lotion are examples of moisturizing cleansers. Some patients like purified micellar water on a cotton ball.

Look out for salicylic acid and niacinamide.
When shopping for skin creams look out for ingredients such as salicylic acid and niacinamide, which will improve your skin's texture, reduce that oil on your skin and help keep the skin feeling smooth. Benzoyl peroxide kills p.acnes bacteria but can also cause dryness – and bleach dark clothing.

> **"** Do not squeeze – it spreads spots and will increase the risk of scarring. **"**

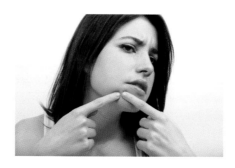

Don't squeeze spots!

Squeezing a spot increases damage to the skin around it. Squeezing spreads inflammation, making your breakouts worse. Our blemish spot gel is one our friends and patients swear by and you can dab it on up to four times a day, even over make-up. Apply it as soon as you see a new acne spot appearing and it will quickly help reduce it.

If you've no products to hand when spots appear, try these DIY helpers.

Crush an aspirin tablet, mix it with water to form a paste and dab it on the spots. Leave it on as long as you can — overnight is ideal. Aspirin is the same medicine as salicylic acid and helps spots heal more quickly.

A blob of toothpaste on a spot will reduce the swelling and so help make it look less angry. It 'draws' the inflamed swelling from the spots.

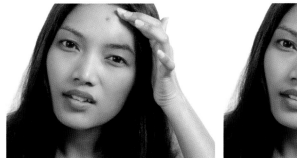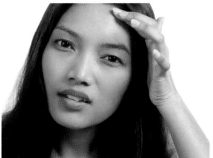

Dab on anti-blemish spot gel at the first sign of a spot — use several times a day.

If you wear caps, hats or headbands

If you wear caps, hats or headbands, the friction against the skin may give you acne on your forehead. If that happens, try applying anti-blemish products to your forehead before putting your cap on.

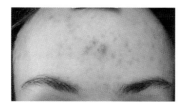

Forehead acne can be caused or made worse by friction from caps, hats and headbands. Apply our day cream with acclenz™ before putting on your headwear.

ACNE AND SUNLIGHT – DOES IT HELP OR HARM?

Sun tan – a quick fix for acne?

Getting a tan is seen by many as a quick fix for acne, but it's just a temporary disguise. It makes it less obvious because the sun causes your skin to redden, tan and camouflage your spots for a few days, but then you may get more blackheads and acne. Tempting as a sun tan may be, it's best to protect from sun.

All skin types need sun protection.

All skin types need sun protection but people with acne-prone skin may find spots get worse if they use thick, high-factor, waterproof sunscreens. Look for oil-free, non-comedogenic formulations, with an SPF of 15 to 30 and with UVA protection (look out for the words 'broad spectrum' on the label).

Only very fair skin needs SPF 50 and only on the sunniest days.

Wear sunhats and clothes that cover you well and stay in the shade, between 11am and 3pm.

If you protect your skin with sun cream you will have less skin-ageing and less risk of skin cancers but you will also make less vitamin D. Take a vitamin D3 supplement, 2000 units each day.

SHOULD YOU SWEAT IT OUT?

Saunas and steam rooms (not to mention DIY steam sessions) are often touted as a way to open the pores and clear skin out. But sweat pores are different from sebaceous pores. The truth is sweating is not going to help. Avoid! It will also give you a red face and eventually lead to thread veins!

CHAPTER 8

MORE SEVERE ACNE

WHEN TO SEEK SPECIALIST HELP AND PRESCRIPTION TREATMENTS

HELP – MY ACNE IS NOT GETTING BETTER

If your acne is not getting better, it's worth going to your GP, who may prescribe prescription treatments or refer you to a dermatologist or a skin specialist physician who will have many more treatment options available. Some of these should be available both on the NHS and privately.

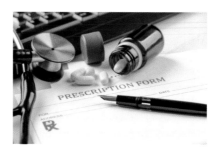

YOU SHOULD SEE A DERMATOLOGIST OR SKIN SPECIALIST PHYSICIAN IF...

you've tried non-prescription, over-the-counter products and not found them effective enough.

your acne is getting worse, leaving scars or red and dark pigmented marks.

your skin is making you feel so unhappy that you're finding it hard to deal with your day-to-day life.

you are embarrassed about your spots and it is affecting your social life and work.

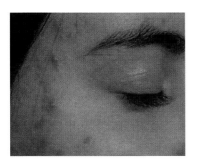 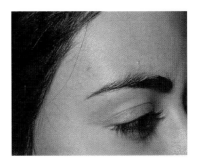

More severe acne before and after an effective acne-treatment programme in our clinic, combining non-prescription and prescription medicines, and our clinic-treatment programme

TOPICAL TREATMENT GELS, LOTIONS AND CREAMS

Topical treatment gels, lotions and creams are usually the first prescriptions for mild to moderate acne. They include a variety of ingredients such as salicylic acid, benzoyl peroxide, niacinamide, azelaic acid, antibiotics and retinoids. They work in different ways, by unplugging pores, by fighting bacteria and by helping skin-cell turnover.

Because they are used at greater strengths than in non-prescription products you may find some irritate your skin, in which case use them less often – say every other night – until your skin is calmer, and use a soap-free moisturizer cleanser, e.g. Aveeno, Cetaphil Lotion, Dermol 500 Lotion or Simple Lotion.

PRESCRIBED RETINOID CREAMS, GELS AND LOTIONS

Topical retinoids should be applied thinly to the whole face, not just on individual spots. Applied this way it will help prevent new spots as well as reduce present ones.

If you are prescribed a retinoid cream or gel, make sure you use it correctly or you will develop red, dry skin.

WHAT ARE RETINOIDS?

RETINOIDS ARE ALL DERIVED FROM THE VITAMIN A MOLECULE.

These are the most frequently prescribed topical retinoids.

Tretinoin cream, gel or lotion
The original anti-acne retinoid, tretinoin can also help improve some signs of ageing skin. In sensitive skin frequent application will cause skin redness and irritation.

Isotretinoin gel
The structure of isotretinoin is slightly different from that of tretinoin and it is less likely to cause irritation. It can be combined with topical antibiotics such as erythromycin. Apply it after washing your face with a moisturizing wash, as the final skin application before bed.

Adapalene gel or cream

Adapalene has the same action as tretinoin and isotretinoin but its activity is more targeted to acne, and less against signs of ageing skin. It is sometimes better tolerated in sensitive skin. It can be combined with antibiotics such as erythromycin.

Tazarotene gel or cream

Tazarotene is a highly effective retinoid for acne. You may find it makes your skin dry, red and flaking if you do not use it exactly according to your doctor's instructions.

Short-contact tazarotene to reduce skin dryness and redness

Apply the tazarotene gel to your skin after a moisturizing lotion wash – see below.

When you use tazarotene leave it on your skin for five minutes – use a timer, and then wash it off with your moisturizing lotion wash in your shower or bath.

You can then gradually increase the time you leave it on if your skin does not get irritated. Some people find they can leave it overnight three or four times a week.

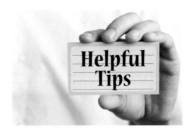

REDUCING YOUR SKIN DRYNESS FROM RETINOID PRODUCTS – SOME FACIAL MOISTURIZING WASHES YOU CAN BUY TO USE WITH YOUR RETINOIDS

Aveeno Facial Wash
Cetaphil Lotion Wash
Dermol 500 Lotion Wash
Simple Facial Wash

Wash with one of these products and a small amount of water, pat (do not rub) your skin dry, and then apply a thin layer of the retinoid.

HOW DO RETINOIDS WORK AGAINST ACNE?

Retinoids all work in the same way. They act on the cells blocking the sebaceous gland ducts enabling them to be shed more easily. Shedding of the cells unblocks the ducts and removes blackheads and whiteheads. Retinoids can help reduce skin discolouration and improve sunken scars by helping the skin to make more collagen to fill the scar.

YOU WILL NOT BE ABLE TO USE RETINOID CREAMS OR GELS IF YOU HAVE VERY SENSITIVE SKIN OR IF YOU HAVE ECZEMA (E.G. ATOPIC ECZEMA) OR HAVE HAD IT IN THE PAST.

IF YOU PLAN TO BECOME PREGNANT YOU SHOULD STOP USING PRESCRIPTION TOPICAL RETINOID.

Retinoids can cause birth defects if used during pregnancy. Even though only small amounts are likely to be absorbed through the skin we feel it wise for you to stop if you become pregnant.

ORAL ANTIBIOTICS

Antibiotic pills may be prescribed to help inflamed acne spots. Antibiotics usually take up to a couple of months to work and are taken until there is no further improvement. Some need to be taken with food, others not, so you need to follow the instructions carefully. Likewise, some antibiotics don't mix well with other medications, such as the contraceptive pill, so check with your physician.

We suggest taking a contraceptive pill in the morning and antibiotic in the early evening with dinner. This minimizes any interaction that might reduce the action of either drug. Doxycycline, tetralysal or minocycline are antibiotics that sometimes cause stomach pain and heartburn. If you are prescribed one of these, to reduce these side effects it's particularly important to take the dose after food in the EARLY evening, NOT just before bed.

Erythromycin, trimethoprim and azithromycin are other antibiotics that can help acne; we try to avoid using these to reduce the risk of antibiotic resistance, that is, the development of strains of bacteria that are not killed by antibiotics. Our acclenz™ Complex products contain no antibiotics.

HORMONE TREATMENT

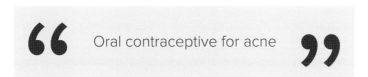

" Oral contraceptive for acne "

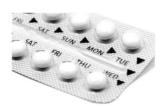

Some contraceptive pills, such as Yaz or Yasmin, can help women with acne, reducing the amount of oil the skin produces by blocking androgen activity. (Other types of contraceptive pill can make acne worse, so do speak to your prescribing physician if your acne is more troublesome than usual.)

Migraine may be caused in some women – or made worse – by oral contraceptives.

Some oral contraceptives carry a risk of causing deep vein thrombosis – blood clots in the veins, which can lead to lung damage and strokes, which can be fatal. Smoking cigarettes will increase these risks – another really good reason to quit smoking!

Spironolactone for acne

Spironolactone has been used for many years as a diuretic tablet to clear excess fluid but it also has good effects for women with acne. It reduces the androgen stimulation of oil glands and works to improve acne. It is usually used together with antibiotics, Roaccutane and oral contraceptives.

POLYCYSTIC OVARIAN SYNDROME (PCOS)

Acne is sometimes a symptom of polycystic ovarian syndrome (PCOS). Other symptoms of this condition include irregular periods and excess facial hair growth and scalp hair thinning. In some women with PCOS blood tests show increased levels of androgen, but in others we find normal androgen levels – it is thought that PCOS acne may result more from the sebaceous glands over-reacting to androgens than from high androgen levels.

Women with PCOS often benefit from seeing both endocrinologists (hormone specialists) and dermatologists. We can do a lot to help control PCOS: we can prescribe medicine to reduce the problems these androgens cause – acne, facial hair growth, hair thinning on your head.

If you have PCOS you may be prescribed oral contraceptives or spironolactone.

ROACCUTANE/ACCUTANE

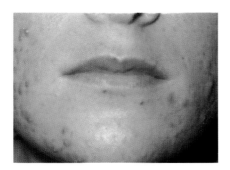 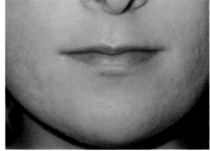

This patient had severe acne and was at risk of post-acne scarring. She had been treated with oral antibiotic and prescription creams for several years. She was then treated with oral Roaccutane treatment and her acne cleared completely.

Oral isotretinoin, (called Roaccutane in the UK and Accutane in USA), is a retinoid taken as pill or capsule. It acts on the oil-producing sebaceous glands and is especially helpful if you have severe acne not helped by other treatments.

However, it is a powerful drug and can only be prescribed by a dermatologist or a physician with extra dermatology training who understands how it works and how to monitor you whilst you are taking it.

We have worked extensively with oral isotretinoin, especially Nick, who started researching it back in 1980.

> " Very severe grade 5 to 6 acne
> may respond to oral Roaccutane
> treatment. "

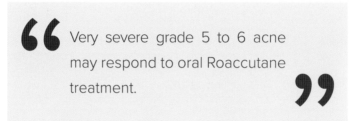

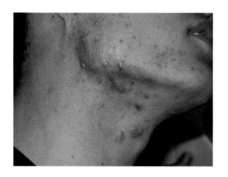

> **"** If you have nodules and cysts you may benefit from a course of Roaccutane. **"**

Oral isotretinoin can harm a foetus.

Because oral isotretinoin can harm a foetus you must not be pregnant when taking this medication.

You must use reliable contraception and have pregnancy tests at monthly intervals.

It is also important that your blood-fat levels and liver functions are tested regularly. If these tests show a change, your dermatologist may change the dose or stop the medication.

What about Roaccutane and depression?

There has been concern that Roaccutane leads to depression. However, recent studies have shown that when some people who took Roaccutane suffered depression and suicidal feelings, it was not the Roaccutane but their severe acne that made them feel desperate and depressed.

We worry about prescribing it to anyone with a history of depression, often suggesting that they see a psychiatrist first.

Our approach with Roaccutane is to start at a low dosage (10mg to 20mg a day), increasing the dose slowly over several months.

This treatment plan can reduce side effects such as dry skin and lips, headaches and muscle ache.

In our experience around 70% of patients remain clear or nearly clear of acne on Roaccutane. Those needing more treatment usually respond better than before Roaccutane – it seems to reset the acne to a less severe level.

> " Your GP may be knowledgeable about acne treatments or will be able to refer you to an NHS specialist.
>
> You can refer yourself to dermatologists and skin specialists physicians privately. "

CHAPTER 9

ACNE IN PREGNANCY

WHY IT HAPPENS AND HOW TO TREAT IT SAFELY

It is difficult to predict if acne will improve or worsen during pregnancy. Some women find they develop acne for the first time during pregnancy.

There are several reasons for this but the change of hormone levels during pregnancy can lead to acne, as discussed in chapter 2.

During the last third of pregnancy, hair becomes oilier due to an increase in sebaceous oil. This increased sebaceous oil can also worsen existing acne and trigger acne in susceptible women.

WHICH TREATMENTS ARE NOT SAFE FOR MOTHER AND FOETUS?

You must not become pregnant if you are on oral Roaccutane. It is safe to conceive three months after stopping.

Other treatments to avoid or stop as soon as you know you are pregnant include oral antibiotics and any hormone-regulating medicines, such as spironolactone or cyproterone.

Any prescription topical retinoid creams or gels should be stopped (even though very small amounts of the medicine of these will be absorbed through the skin) as it is thought that these can affect the developing child.

Topical antibiotics except erythromycin gel or lotion should be stopped if you know you are pregnant. Other treatments that we do not advise during pregnancy include skin peels containing salicylic acid or retinoic acid, intense pulse lights and lasers.

Benzoyl peroxide is considered safe during pregnancy, although no formal research has been reported.

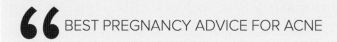

BEST PREGNANCY ADVICE FOR ACNE

If you know you are (or think you may be) pregnant, stop all prescription treatments until you have discussed the situation with your dermatologist or general practitioner.

They can guide you on safe treatments for acne during your pregnancy.

TREATMENTS FOR ACNE THAT CAN BE USED DURING PREGNANCY

Most non-prescription creams and gels with the exception of those that contain high levels of salicylic acid can be used.

Topical erythromycin gel or lotion can be used.

It is wise to apply creams and gels to small areas, for example, just the face, and not to apply over large areas of your chest and back. This keeps absorption of the ingredients to a minimum.

CLINIC TREATMENTS FOR ACNE THAT CAN BE USED DURING PREGNANCY

Make sure the clinic knows about your pregnancy. Safe treatments include some fruit acid peels, e.g. glycolic acid or lactic acid.

Dermasweep and other forms of microdermabrasion are safe but we avoid solutions that contain ingredients such as salicylic acid, skin lightening preparations and retinoids.

Steam and extraction by medical therapists can be very helpful.

If you get larger painful, and potentially scarring, spots and nodules, it is safe to have them injected with dilute cortisone (see chapter 10).

WHAT ABOUT ACNE TREATMENTS AFTER PREGNANCY?

Non-prescription treatments including our products are safe to continue. All the active ingredients are at low, safe, levels in the products.

Treatments that are safe during breastfeeding include prescription antibiotic creams and gels, such as erythromycin, benzoyl peroxide, and topical retinoid gels and creams. But, again, apply to a small area only, such as the face.

If you are breastfeeding, avoid taking medicines by mouth that are absorbed into the body and into your milk. Examples are oral erythromycin, tetracyclines and minocycline.

If you are not breastfeeding then it is safe to resume all the options listed previously in chapters 7, 8 and 9.

It is also safe to resume stronger peels containing salicylic acid at the clinic, and, if you have red inflamed acne, to have treatments with lasers and intense pulsed light to reduce the redness and risk of scarring.

Pregnancy is a wonderful time for most women, but having acne during pregnancy can be a frustrating and occasionally painful experience.

TREATMENTS DURING PREGNANCY

Safe during pregnancy	Avoid during pregnancy
Most non-prescription creams and gels	Retinoid creams and gels
Erythromycin lotion and gel	Salicylic acid peels
Glycolic Acid peels	Retinoid peels
Lactic Acid peels	Most oral antibiotics
Steam and Extraction	Most antibiotic creams or gels
Microdermabrasion	Roaccutane
Injection of cortisone into larger spots	

CHAPTER 10

ACNE TREATMENTS AT THE CLINIC

WE HAVE SEVERAL TREATMENTS IN OUR CLINIC TO HELP ACNE

Treatments in our clinic can improve active blemishes and help to minimize scarring. They also help to speed up the improvement from your non-prescription or prescription treatments.

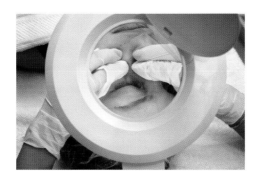

> **66** Our dermatology-trained nurses and therapists treat acne and comedones with steam and extraction. Other techniques we use include microdermabrasion, vacuum and visible light (Isolaz) and peels. **99**

EXTRACTION AND STEAM CLEANSING

Our nurses and therapists gently remove blocked acne spots, blackheads and whiteheads with gloved fingers.

DERMASWEEP – SUCTION MICRODERMABRASION

This is a gentle, superficial dermabrasion, which helps to extract the comedones by suction. Immediately after suction we apply an anti-acne solution, which is quickly absorbed into the skin. The type of solution is selected for your type of skin and acne.

ANTI-ACNE CHEMICAL PEELS

We use different solutions to help your acne; these gently peel off dead skin cells and help to unblock pores. Peel solutions contain various anti-acne ingredients, including lactic acid, salicylic acid, glycolic acid and resorcinol.

LASER AND INTENSE-PULSED-LIGHTS TREATMENTS

Laser and intense-pulsed-lights treatments can be very effective in reducing the redness of acne and acne scars. The lasers are absorbed by the red blood cells and reduce blood flow in any red spots.

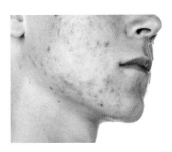

> **66** Laser and filtered intense-pulsed-lights treatments can reduce red inflamed acne lesions and scars. **99**

INJECTION OF DILUTE CORTISONE

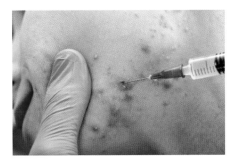

Painful, inflamed spots and larger acne bumps can be cleared with the help of an injection of dilute cortisone. Make sure that you receive this treatment from a trained skin physician or dermatologist, as too big a dose or too deep an injection can leave a hollow.

VISIBLE LIGHT TREATMENTS

Acne bacteria produce a chemical that is absorbed by blue and red visible light. Light activation of this chemical kills the acne bacteria. Our clinic uses Isolaz, which uses vacuum suction to 'pull' the acne spots closer to the light, which then kills the bacteria and reduces the spots.

PHOTODYNAMIC THERAPY (PDT) AND SEVERE ACNE

Photodynamic therapy is a treatment for more severe acne. After prescription lotion or gel has been applied, the treated skin is exposed in a controlled way to visible light or sunlight to 'activate' the medicine. This treatment has to be directed by dermatologist familiar with PDT.

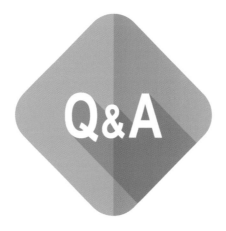

QUESTIONS AND ANSWERS ABOUT YOUR ACNE

Q: Does darker skin need different acne treatment to pale skin?

A: (Nick) Acne treatments are fairly similar for both skin types, but there are some differences that need to be considered. In darker skin types there's a higher risk of post-acne hyperpigmentation, that is, dark marks where the blemishes have been. Prescription retinoid creams work on the acne and lightening creams on the pigmentation.

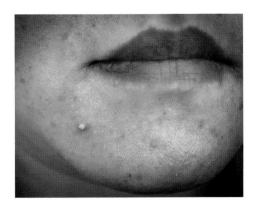

Red acne spots can become darker in darker skin types.

It's fine to use some over-the-counter acne skincare with ingredients such as salicylic acid, witch hazel and niacinamide; this helps dark marks – see our **acclenz**™ Complex for these ingredients.

Q: I have spots, but want to wear make-up. Will it make things worse?

A: (Philippa) Heavy make-up may clog pores. You can get caught in a vicious circle of applying more make-up to cover up blemished skin. So, if you want to wear foundation, check that it is oil-free and labelled non-comedogenic.

Mineral powder foundation works really well for lots of people and doesn't seem to cause breakouts. It also minimizes shine and doesn't irritate the skin.

Apply an anti-acne product, like our Anti-Blemish Serum, before make-up.

> **"** Good camouflage make-up can really help you mask your spots until they can be cleared. **"**

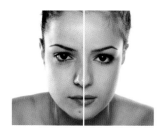

Q: Does keeping skin squeaky clean help guard against breakouts?

A: (Nick) It's a good idea to keep skin as clean as possible by cleansing morning and evening. However, 'squeaky clean' sounds like over-cleansing to me. The danger with this is that you can dry your skin out, especially if you are also using acne medications. If your skin is oily you probably think you'd like to dry your skin out, but this is not the right approach. Go for a gentle cleanser, e.g., a lotion plus an oil-reducing cream and cleanser, or micellar water. Soaps and astringent toners are best avoided as they over-strip the skin of its oils.

Q: What causes spots before a period?

A: (Philippa) These are due to changing hormone levels. Just before your period you have a change in progesterone and oestrogens ratios, which causes breakouts. If you already on anti-acne medication, increase your dose the week before your period – and have your spot-gel handy.

CHAPTER 11

HELP! I HAVE ACNE SCARS

IMPROVING ACNE SCARS

We have a variety of treatments to help reduce different types of scars — fillers, lasers, radio-frequency systems and injections. We will guide you through these various scars and the treatments.

> **"** Try not to squeeze or pick acne! It can create acne scars. **"**

If you have this habit, try to retrain yourself by dabbing spot-gel on any new or existing spots. This may help you resist the temptation to squeeze and scratch at the spot.

MEDICAL NAMES FOR DIFFERENT TYPES OF SCARS CAUSED BY ACNE

Erythematous	Red scars
Hypertrophic	Thick scars
Keloid	Very thick scars
Atrophic	Sunken, hollow rolling scars
Ice pick	Small deep scars
Hyper-pigmented	Dark scars
Hypo-pigmented	Light scars

ERYTHEMATOUS (RED) SCARS

Erythematous scars often remain after acne spots have cleared. They may fade over time or in some cases result in sunken scars.

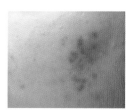

Red scars following acne

ATROPHIC SCARS

Inflamed acne can produce sunken scars as a result of damage to the skin's support tissues — collagen and elastin. These sunken types of scars are called atrophic scars. Deep small scars are called ice pick scars.

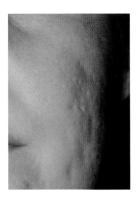

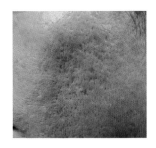

Atrophic rolling scars may occur on the cheeks after acne nodules and cysts.

Deep ice pick scars usually occur on cheeks after multiple inflamed spots on the cheeks.

HYPERTROPHIC AND KELOID SCARS

In some people inflammation causes the opposite type of scar from the sunken, atrophic, one: hypertrophic or keloid scars, which are red, raised, thickened scars, more common on the jaw line, lower face, neck and upper body.

You may have a risk of developing thickened scars after skin injury and surgery. They are caused by overproduction of collagen, which is made in skin cells called fibroblasts.

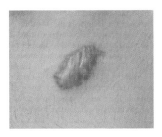

Thick keloid scars, which can occur after more inflamed acne spots

SCARS IN PIGMENTED SKIN

Acne in olive and darker skin types will go from redness to darkening. We call this hyperpigmentation.

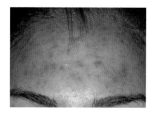

Acne may result in skin darkening from inflamed spots in a person with darker skin.

DIFFERENT SCARS NEED DIFFERENT TREATMENTS

If your scars are red, laser or intense-pulsed-light (IPL) can help to improve them and calm inflamed spots too.

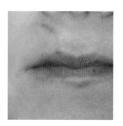 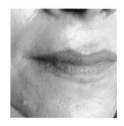

Red scars on upper lip: before and after vascular laser treatments

SUNKEN ATROPHIC SCARS: OPTIONS

Subcision – using a needle or micro-blade to cut through fibrous scar tissues under the scar, allowing skin surface to rise
Fillers into the scar to raise them – Hyaluronic Acid, or Ellanse Sculptra
Fraxel Laser, tightening and lifting scars
Fractional Radio-frequency (RF), tightening and lifting scars – safe for darker skin types

For localized sunken scars, we use an injectable filler containing hyaluronic acid.

When there are many sunken scars, an injected filler called Sculptra stimulates the skin to produce its own collagen to fill out the scars.

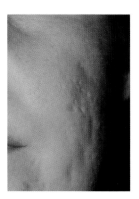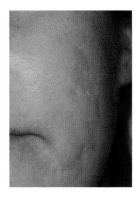

Sunken scars on cheeks: before and after four treatment sessions with subcision and Sculptra injection followed by fractional radiofrequency

For multiple rolling hollow scars, Fraxel repair carbon dioxide laser, sometimes combined with radiofrequency, tightens the skin around the scar, making the skin surface more even.

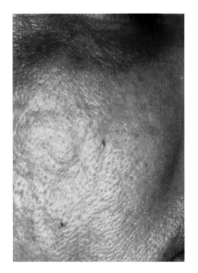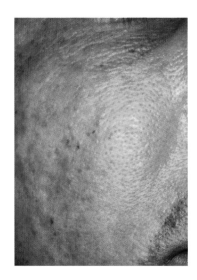

Rolling hollow scars on the cheeks of a patient: before and after fractional carbon dioxide lasers and radiofrequency

For many punched out and ice pick scars, fractional micro needle radiofrequency is able to tighten the skin around scars making the skin smoother and scars less severe. It can also be used on any skin colour.

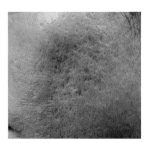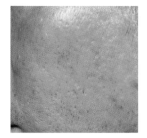

Multiple punched out and ice-pick scars: before and after four treatment sessions of Intracel micro radiofrequency

Thick, raised, keloid scars can be injected with cortisone or other medicines by a specialist physician or dermatologist. We can improve these with fractional laser or radiofrequency followed by strong cortisone cream to reduce the scar thickness. The laser helps the cortisone cream to penetrate into the thick scars.

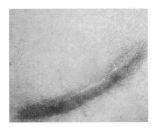 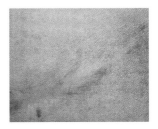

Thick raised keloid scars after acne cyst on shoulder: before and after cortisone injections and Fraxel carbon dioxide laser

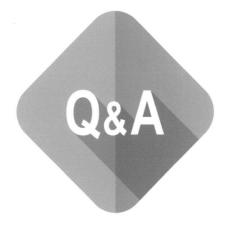

Q: My acne has left me with red scars. Is there anything that can help?

A: (Nick) When scarring is red but isn't too deep, you can try an anti-redness cream at home with ingredients such as antioxidants, niacinamide and chamomile, which will calm and soothe the skin.

A vascular laser or intense-pulsed-light can be very effective.

CHAPTER 12

KNOW YOUR INGREDIENTS

NON-PRESCRIPTION ANTI-ACNE PRODUCTS

---

acclenz™ Complex

Patent-pending, anti-blemish complex of six different ingredient groups, shown to kill all tested strains of acne bacteria, including some resistant to antibiotics. It improves blemishes in subjects with acne and causes no skin dryness or irritancy.

Allantoin

A skin-soothing agent that reduces skin redness from inflammation, moisturizes and helps repair damaged skin.

Antioxidants

Antioxidants reduce inflammation; they also reduce the damage caused to your skin by acne by reducing the harmful free radicals produced by inflammation. Antioxidants used in anti-acne products include acai extract, ascorbyl palmitate, blueberry extract, ferrulic acid, goji extract, retinyl palmitate, tocopherol acetate and vitamins A, C and E.

Benzoyl peroxide (BPO)

BPO is used both on prescription and in non-prescription products. Antimicrobial and comedolytic, it can be combined with oral or topical antibiotics and retinoids. Side effects can be a problem and include bleaching of hair, clothes and bedding and skin irritancy. For this reason it's advisable to use BPO at the lowest strength (e.g. 2.5%) at first, slowly increasing the strength only if necessary.

Bisobolol

The active skin-calming ingredient in bisobolol is chamomile extract. It is useful for inflamed irritated skin.

Chamomile extract

A botanical agent that reduces skin redness and irritation, chamomile is very useful for targeting inflammation of acne and skin irritation plus redness resulting from retinoid application. It is an ingredient in our acclenz™ Complex.

Chlorhexidine

Chlorhexidine is a powerful antiseptic and antibacterial; it is effective, without causing sensitivity issues, at very dilute levels. It is an ingredient in our acclenz™ Complex

Eucalyptus extract

A botanical antiseptic, eucalyptus extract has anti-blemish action and is active against acne-causing bacteria. It is an ingredient in our acclenz™ Complex.

Glycerin

Glycerin is a humectant; it moisturizes and improves skin softness, reduces dryness and scaliness and helps repair the skin barrier when it becomes damaged

Hyaluronate and hyaluronic acid

Like glycerin, hyaluronate and hyaluronic acid are humectants, and their actions are similar to those of glycerin.

Niacinamide

Niacinamide has numerous beneficial effects on skin: it is anti-inflammatory, it normalizes skin-cell development, it reduces red blemishes, it repairs damage to the skin barrier, it reduces scaling and skin sensitivity, and it reduces post-acne pigmented dark patches. It is an ingredient in our acclenz™ Complex.

Pyrolidone Carboxylic Acid (PCA)

PCA helps to repair the skin barrier damaged by acne inflammation. It is combined with zinc in our acclenz™ Complex.

Retinoids (non-prescription strength)

Related to vitamin A in structure, the retinoids retinol, retinaldehyde and retinyl palmitate stimulate the skin to shed dead cells, (which helps reduce blackheads) and to grow new healthy outer skin.

Salicylic acid

Salicylic acid reduces blemishes by stimulating the shedding of pore-plugging comedones, and blemished skin. It also reduces redness and boosts the beneficial effects of retinoids. It is an ingredient in our acclenz™ Complex.

Sulphur

Sulphur has been used for many years to calm inflamed acne and help reduce skin surface oil.

Vitamin A

Vitamin A is the precursor of retinoids. For the action of vitamin A, see 'Retinoids'.

Willow bark

Willow bark is a botanical source of salicylic acid. Its actions are the same as for synthetic salicylic acid but concentration of the active ingredient in samples of the botanical extract will vary. Willow bark is an ingredient in our acclenz™ Complex.

Zinc

Zinc is anti-seborrheic, (that is, it reduces sebum oil) and anti-bacterial. It is combined with PCA in our acclenz™ Complex.

CHAPTER 13

KNOW YOUR INGREDIENTS

PRESCRIPTION MEDICINES FOR ACNE

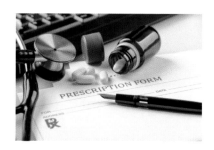

RETINOIDS – PRESCRIPTION

TRETINOIN, ISOTRETINOIN, ADAPALENE, TAZAROTENE

Retinoids are products developed from vitamin A; they have comedolytic and anti-inflammatory effects. They can be used alone to treat acne but are best combined with an antibiotic or non-irritating products to reduce their potential for skin irritation.

ANTIBIOTICS

ANTIBIOTICS HAVE BOTH ANTIMICROBIAL AND
ANTI-INFLAMMATORY EFFECTS. THEY CAN BE
TOPICAL OR BE TAKEN BY MOUTH.

Topical antibiotics

Topical antibiotics are ideal for patients with mild to moderate acne, but they do not reduce comedones. They can be used in combination with a retinoid, with benzoyl peroxide or with our new acclenz™ containing product.

Antibiotics by mouth – oral antibiotics

Oral antibiotics have the same action as topical antibiotics but the oral route is more effective and practical for diffuse, widespread acne, including acne on the back. Antibiotics have more anti-inflammatory power when taken orally.

AZELAIC ACID

Patients who cannot tolerate topical retinoids or benzoyl peroxide may benefit from azelaic acid cream or gel as it is less irritating. It also helps lighten post-acne dark skin patches and scars.

DAPSONE

Dapsone has an anti-inflammatory effect by mouth. It is not an oral antibiotic or as effective as isotretinoin but may be used in cases when isotretinoin is contraindicated. Patients with a particular type of anaemia cannot be treated with Dapsone. In the USA a topical Dapsone gel has been developed.

CORTICOSTEROIDS AND CORTISONES

Corticosteroids injections can be very helpful in clearing large, painful, potentially scarring spots. Corticosteroids also help to reduce hypertrophic and keloid post-acne scars.

ORAL ISOTRETINOIN (ROACCUTANE OR ACCUTANE)

See chapter 8 for a detailed account of the benefits and side effects of oral isotretinoin, which is sold under the names Roaccutane in the UK and Accutane in the USA.

Oral isotretinoin is reserved for more severe acne that has failed to respond to other treatments. 70% of people treated with oral isotretinoin have long-term clearance.

> " Isotretinion, like other retinoids, is teratogenic, that is, it harms the foetus. It must not be taken if you are pregnant or actively trying for pregnancy. "

ANDROGEN-BLOCKING MEDICINES

ORAL CONTRACEPTIVE PILLS

These medications have sebum-reducing effects. Side effects include increased risk of thromboembolic disease (clots in veins and lungs), migraine and stroke, especially in smokers. Yaz, Yasmin and Dianette are contraceptive pills that are often prescribed as anti-acne treatment.

SPIRONOLACTONE

Spironolactone was originally developed as a diuretic (a tablet taken to reduce water retention) and to control high blood pressure but it has anti-androgen effects on sebaceous glands and acne. It is often effective in women for acne, oily skin, excess hair growth and polycystic ovarian syndrome.

CHAPTER 14

PHYSICIANS AND OTHERS WHO CAN HELP WITH YOUR ACNE

OTHERS WHO CLAIM THEY CAN –

WHO ARE THEY? WHAT IS THEIR TRAINING?

There are many 'therapists' and skin-care 'professionals' who will claim to be able to treat your spots and acne. Many will not, in our opinion, have had sufficient training to justify their claims – or, indeed, any at all.

Some examples: some nurses, beauty therapists, medical assistants, chiropractors, cosmetologists, hairdressers and pharmacists will offer to help you with your acne. But they may not have the training or experience to provide you with reliable care.

> **""** Do not be afraid to ask about the background and training of someone offering you advice. **""**

GENERAL PRACTITIONER

In the UK your GP will have had three years' training in general practice after medical school. A GP *may* be knowledgeable about skin diseases and treatments *if* they have also taken additional dermatology training after GP training. In this case they will be described as a GP with special interest in the skin or a skin specialist physician.

Unfortunately, many medical students have only a week or less of dermatology training; as a result some GPs may not always be confident with dermatology problems and treatments.

SPECIALIST PHYSICIAN IN SKIN

Specialist physicians in skin are doctors who after their medical school training take additional intensive training, and gain experience, in dermatology. Some will have also had extra training in cosmetic procedures, such as laser, filler and other treatments for scars.

Philippa, is such a doctor. 'After six years at medical school and three years' hospital training, I spent more than ten years working at the Cranley Clinic, gaining valuable dermatology experience, directing numerous research programmes and publishing them in scientific journals. I then took an extra year of education and training in dermatology, passing the examination for the Diploma in Dermatology.'

DERMATOLOGIST

A dermatologist in the UK will have had at least four years of specialist internal medicine training after medical school.

After passing the examinations for the Royal College of Physicians, they are allowed to apply for dermatology training. They will spend another five to six years as dermatology trainees. This means a combined total of nine to ten years of internal medicine and dermatology training after five to six years at medical school – a total of up to sixteen years of training.

Dermatologists are the ultimate experts for all skin, hair and nail diseases.

Some take extra training in skin surgery and cosmetic procedures (Nick did this in the USA) and are experts in other treatments you may need, for example, lasers, fillers and scar treatments, and in skin cancers and skin rejuvenation.

Unfortunately for the UK, because of poor government decisions and a lack of training positions, there are too few dermatologists being trained in this country.

The UK has only one tenth of the dermatologists for the size of its population that France, Germany, Italy, Spain, the USA and Canada have – approximately 650 in the UK compared, (for example), with 5,000 in France, for a similar population size.

Unfortunately it is likely that, in the future, UK dermatology training – currently one of the most intensive in the world – will be reduced.

REGISTERED NURSE AND NURSE PRACTITIONER

Some registered nurses and nurse practitioners, for example our clinic nurses, will have acquired additional dermatology skills after nursing school training; they will have learnt about skin treatments, including those for acne, and about lasers, hair removal and peels.

BEAUTY THERAPIST

Some beauty therapists, such as the medical aestheticians in our clinic, have had extra training in various clinic treatments and are extremely skilled in treating patients undertaking our clinic acne programme.

THE STAFF AT OUR CLINIC INCLUDE

a dermatologist
a skin specialist physician
a registered general nurse (RGN)
a medical aesthetician
research assistants
clinical administrators

WE OFFER THE FOLLOWING ACNE TREATMENTS:

Dermasweep microdermabrasion
peels
steam and extraction
Isolaz
lasers
pulsed lights
visible light and photodynamic therapy
Acne scar treatments with prescription and non-prescription medication

ABOUT THE AUTHORS
WHO ARE WE?

We are a dermatologist (Nick) and skin specialist physician, (Philippa), who have been caring for patients with skin problems for many years in both the UK and the USA.

We frequently see the frustration, emotional and physical discomfort that acne and blemishes cause. We have developed treatment programmes tailored to different types of acne, different skin types and completely new, effective, products and treatments.

DR NICK LOWE, M.B., CH.B., M.D., F.R.C.P, F.A.C.P., CONSULTANT DERMATOLOGIST AND PROFESSOR OF DERMATOLOGY

I am a consultant dermatologist in London and Clinical Professor of Dermatology at UCLA School of Medicine in Los Angeles, California.

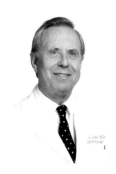

I studied medicine at the University of Liverpool and then volunteered as a doctor in the Royal Navy, training as an internal medicine specialist at the main Royal Navy Hospital.

I did dermatology training at the University of Southampton, the University of Liverpool, and then as a fellow at Scripps Clinic in California and the University of California, San Diego.

After the fellowship I wanted to continue dermatology research and I was fortunate in being able to stay in the USA.

I became Professor of Dermatology at UCLA School of Medicine, seeing patients, training dermatologists and developing treatment programmes in lasers, phototherapy and psoriasis treatment, as well as directing a varied research programme.

Some of my research at that time was about the effects of vitamin A compounds (retinoids) on the skin, highly effective treatments for acne and skin rejuvenation.

In 1994, when our daughter Philippa started at medical school in England, I founded the Cranley Clinic in London, modelled on my California Dermatology Centre. This proved to be very successful and it is great to be able to work with Philippa.

I am a great believer in education, and in scientific research, and have published over 450 clinical and research papers, and scientific publications. This will be the twentieth book that I have written for my peers or for the public.

I am so fortunate to have been a dermatologist during the era of new, highly effective treatments for many skin diseases, including acne over the last three decades.

We want with this book to share the knowledge gained over our combined years of experience to help those with acne.

DR PHILIPPA LOWE, M.B., CH.B., DIPLOMA OF LAW, DIPLOMA IN DERMATOLOGY, SPECIALIST PHYSICIAN IN SKIN

Growing up in California seeing the enthusiasm and knowledge of my dermatologist dad gave me a natural inclination to learn more about the skin and skin diseases, of which one of the most frequent and important is acne.

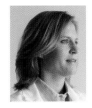

I lived in California until I was eighteen years old, when I graduated from Santa Monica High School and started as an undergraduate at the University of California at Berkeley. But I was offered a place at the University of Liverpool Medical School, accepted it and graduated with Dean's commendation in 1998.

My specialty training was interrupted by three delightful children, Annie, Charlie and Tom. I took a law course, graduating with a postgraduate diploma in law. This gave me insight into medical ethics and the ethical treatment of our patients.

I have worked at the Cranley Clinic and Research Centre in London for over ten years, treating patients, conducting research and working in our acne clinic.

Two years ago I specialized further and completed the Diploma in Dermatology at The Royal London and St Bartholomew's hospitals.

With our combined experiences and knowledge we are able to offer the highest quality skin care. I share my dad's desire to help to educate and guide people with acne to obtain the best information and treatment.

ACKNOWLEDGEMENTS

We wish to thank all our patients for entrusting their skin problems to us, and our clinic staff for being so supportive to us and caring towards our patients.

We would like to thank our administration staff, particularly Emily and Linda, for their help with this manuscript.

And we'd like to thank our family, particularly Pam, Nick's wife and Philippa's mother, for her support and advice, and Philippa's husband, Mike, and three children, Annie, Charlie and Tom, for giving Philippa time for this book.

GLOSSARY

Acai extract:
An *antioxidant* extract from the acai fruit

Accutane:
Brand name (used in the USA) of *isotretinoin*, a powerful prescription-only oral medicine derived from *vitamin A* and used to treat severe acne

Adapalene:
A prescription-only medicine (brand name *Differin*) derived from *vitamin A* and used as a *topical* treatment for acne

Adrenal glands:
Glands that produce a variety of different *hormones*, including *cortisol* and *androgens* (both of which may lead to a worsening of acne)

Allantoin:
A skin-soothing ingredient of skin creams for sensitive skin

Amino acid:
A building block for proteins in the body including the skin

Androgens:
Hormones that are produced in adolescence and during adult life, more in males than females, responsible for body maturation – sometimes lead to acne and excessive hair growth

Anti-androgen:
A medicine that reduces the effects of *androgens*

Antibiotics (or antibacterials)
Type of *antimicrobial* used in the treatment and prevention of bacterial infection

Antibiotic resistance:
The development of strains of bacteria that are not harmed by the *antibiotics* that used to be effective against that type of organism

Antiepileptic medicines:
Medicines that help control epileptic seizures. One such medicine, phenobarbitone, sometimes has the side effect of causing acne

Anti-inflammatory:
Having the effect of reducing redness or inflammation in the skin and body

Antioxidant:
Substances that neutralize the potential of *free radicals* to cause harmful effects

Anti-seborrhoeic:
Having the effect of reducing the activity or output of *sebaceous glands*

Antidepressants:
Medications that reduce depression

Antimicrobial:
Having the effect of reducing bacteria and other micro-organisms, for example yeast

Antiseptic:
Antimicrobial

Ascorbyl palmitate:
A chemically stable form of *vitamin C* used in skin preparations

Atrophic scar:
A scar resulting from thinning of the skin tissue

Azelaic acid:
A medication that can be helpful for acne and *rosacea*, typical trade names are Finacea and Skinoren

Azithromycin:
One of the oral *antibiotics*

Benzoyl peroxide:
An anti-acne ingredient in non-prescription and some prescription products

Beta-hydroxy acids:
A group of chemicals used in skin cream of which *salicylic acid* is a member

Bisabolol:
An extract of the *chamomile* plant with excellent skin-calming activity

Blood-vessel-targeted lasers:
Laser light that is absorbed by the red blood cells in the blood vessels. These lasers are used to reduce the redness of some acne scars, and multiple thread veins. They are also helpful for *rosacea* treatment

Blueberry extract:
An *antioxidant* extract from blueberries

BPO:
Abbreviation for **benzoyl peroxide**

Broad spectrum:
Giving sunscreen protection from different wavelengths of sunlight, both ultraviolet B and ultraviolet A (**UVA**)

Carbohydrates, complex:
Complex carbohydrates are composed of complex molecules. These need to be broken down by the body and their nutrients are only slowly and gradually released into the bloodstream. They are found in foods such as wholegrain wheat and brown rice, and usually contain nutrients other than sugar, such as fibre, vitamins and minerals

Carbohydrates, simple:
Simple carbohydrates are composed of simple molecules that are easily broken down by the body. The sugar and glucose they contain are rapidly absorbed, and can cause damage to the skin and a worsening of acne

Carbon dioxide (CO2):
A naturally occurring gas (present in air) used in **laser** treatment. We breathe out carbon dioxide

Chamomile:
See **bisabolol**

Chlorhexidine:
An **antimicrobial** ingredient used in washes and creams

Cholesterol:
A type of fat that is present in many tissues including blood and skin

CO2 (sometimes written as CO_2):
Carbon dioxide

Collagen:
One of the components of the tissue that gives skin support and structure

Comedogenic:
Likely to cause an increase in **comedones**, the first stage of acne

Comedolytic:
Likely to reduce **comedones**

Comedones:
Whiteheads and blackheads (formed by plugging of the opening of the **sebaceous oil ducts**) – the first stage of acne

Corticosteroids:
Medications (similar in structure to some **hormones** produced by the body) used to reduce the effects of inflammation

Cortisol:
A type of **corticosteroid**

Cortisone:
A type of **corticosteroid** (also a natural **hormone** produced by the body)

Cosmetic procedure:
A treatment intended to improve the overall appearances of a person

Cyproterone:
An **anti-androgen** commonly included in some contraceptive pills

Cyst:
Sac – or small enclosed cavity – often fluid-filled. Cysts occur in acne when inflammation causes damage to the skin and enlargement of a spot

Dapsone:
An anti-inflammatory medicine used for different types of acne, taken by mouth or applied to the skin

Deep vein thrombosis (DVT):
Formation of blood clots in the veins – usually of the legs, but sometimes in other parts of the body. Some oral contraceptives may increase the incidence of DVT

Dermabrasion:
A superficial procedure to remove outer skin cells

DermaSweep:
A vacuum-assisted technique of ***dermabrasion***

Dermatologist:
A physician trained in all aspects of diagnosis and treatment of skin, hair, and nails

Dermatology:
The branch of medicine relating to skin, hair and nails

Dianette:
One oral contraceptive pill containing the ***anti-androgen cyproterone***

Differin cream and gel:
Preparations containing ***adapalene***

Diuretic:
A tablet that reduces excessive build-up of fluid and water in the body

Doxycycline:
One of the ***antibiotics*** that can be used for acne treatment

DVT:
Abbreviation for ***deep vein thrombosis***

Elastin:
A protein in the skin enabling it to be elastic

Endocrinologist:
A physician specializing in understanding ***hormones***

Endorphins:
Chemicals released by the body during activities such as exercise. Endorphins are often called 'feel-good' ***hormones*** and are thought to improve health and general quality of life

Epidermis:
The outermost part of the skin, made up of many layers of cells, which forms a protective barrier

Erythematous:
Having a red or inflamed appearance

Erythromycin:
One of the ***antibiotics*** used to treat acne. It can be taken by mouth or applied as a cream or gel

Ethical:
Appropriately professional and caring

Exfoliation:
Gently removal of the dead cells from the skin surface

Fatty acids:
Chemical components of fats such as ***cholesterol*** and ***sebaceous oil***

Ferulic acid:
A highly effective *antioxidant* used in skin-care products

Fibroblast:
Cells in the skin that produce *collagen* and *elastin* and assist skin healing after injury

Fillers:
Injectable substances that can help with skin wrinkles and scars. Most fillers contain *hyaluronic acid*

Flavonoids:
A group of *antioxidant* structures present in some foods, for example green tea

Foetus:
Unborn child

Fractional RF:
Radiofrequency delivered by tiny needles to assist in skin *rejuvenation* and improvement of acne scars

Fraxel Repair CO2 laser:
Laser that delivers its energy through microscopic, grid-like, holes. This enables the skin to heal much more quickly than after other types of CO2 laser. Fraxel Repair CO2 Laser is a make of *fractional laser*

Free radicals:
Unstable chemicals (produced as a result of a variety of insults to the skin and other tissue, for example, environmental pollution, tobacco smoke and sunlight exposure) which cause damage to body cells by the process of *oxidation*

Glycaemic Index:
A rating system for ***carbohydrate*** foods showing how quickly each food affects the blood sugar level

Glycerine:
An ingredient used in many moisturizers because it is a humectant, that is, it attracts and holds moisture in the skin

Glycolic acid:
A substance derived from apples used to help remove dead skin cells from the skin surface

Goji extract:
An ***antioxidant*** extracted from the goji fruit

Hormones:
Chemicals released from the body that affect and help various body actions

Hyaluronic acid:
One of the building blocks of ***collagen*** – the most important ingredient in skin-filling injections to reduce wrinkles and hollow scars

Hydrocortisone:
A ***corticosteroid*** commonly used in creams to reduce skin redness and inflammation

Hyperpigmentation:
Increased darkening of the skin

Hypertrophic scar:
A scar resulting from thickening of part of the skin

Insulin:
A ***hormone*** responsible for regulating levels of blood sugar

Intense pulsed light treatment:
A high-powered light source with filters to select different wavelengths of light, used for improvement of skin redness and discolouration, useful for acne, *rosacea* and red scars

INTRAcel:
One of the manufacturers of *fractional radiofrequency*

IPL:
Abbreviation for *intense pulsed light*

Isolase:
A form of treatment using visible light and suction to reduce blackheads and whiteheads

Isotretinoin:
The pharmacologic name for *Accutane*

Isotrex:
Gel preparation containing isotretinoin

Isotrexin:
Gel preparation containing *isotretinoin* and *erythromycin*

Keloid scar:
A *hypertrophic scar* that is larger than the original *lesion*

Lactic acid:
A milder version (derived from milk) of the active constituent in *glycolic acid*

Laser:
A single wavelength of light that can be used in *dermatology* to target various skin problems including redness, darkness and scars

Lesion:
In *dermatology*, any skin spot or blemish

Lipids:
Scientific term for fats and oils

Lithium:
A drug used for depression and manic-depressive illness

Lycopene:
An *antioxidant* derived from various vegetables, including tomatoes

Lymecyline
See *Tetralysal*

Melatonin:
A *hormone* naturally present in the body that helps the 'body clock' maintain day-time/night-time rhythms

Metronidazole:
An *antibiotic* medicine used in the treatment of *rosacea* and sometimes inflamed acne

Micellar water:
A cleansing water used on a cotton ball for sensitive skin

Microneedles:
Microscopically small needles used, for example, in *fractional radiofrequency*

Microdermabrasion:
Gentle surface *exfoliation* with a *dermabrasion* machine

Microspheres:
Tiny spheres containing minute quantities of a medication. Formulation

of a medication using microspheres enables its slow, controlled release into the tissues it is being used to treat

Mineral powder:
Make-up powder that tends to contain fewer potential skin irritants, e.g., preservatives, chemical dyes, fragrance

Minocycline:
An *antibiotic* taken by mouth, useful for acne and rosacea

Niacin:
One form of *vitamin B3*, helpful in regulating the skin's function as a protection barrier and in reducing inflammation and discolouration from acne. It is available in creams and as an oral supplement

Niacinamide:
Another form of *vitamin B3*

Nodules:
Larger lumps on the skin

Non-comedogenic:
Not an acne-trigger when applied to the skin

Occlusion:
Blockage

Oestrogens:
The *hormones* that regulate various body functions in women, e.g., menstruation and maintenance of pregnancy

Oral:
Taken by mouth

Oxidation:
The process by which **free radicals** cause body cells to be changed chemically, and gradually to lose proper functionality

Panthenol:
Vitamin B5

PCA:
Pyrrolidone carboxylic acid, an important skin chemical that forms the skin barrier

Peel:
Solution applied to the skin that make the dead cells on the surface peel off

Propionibacterium acnes (p. acnes):
The bacteria that cause inflammation in acne spots

Psoriasis:
A common skin disease characterized by redness and scaling of the skin – usually in patches on the knees and elbows, but sometimes elsewhere on the body

Radiofrequency:
A type of energy used medicinally

Radiofrequency systems:
A treatment that uses **radiofrequency** to the skin to reduce hollow post-acne scars by stimulating the production of **collagen**

Rejuvenation:
The process of becoming or being made more youthful

Resorcinol:
One of the ingredients of a common chemical peel – often used together with **salicylic acid** and **lactic acid**

Retinaldehyde:
A type of *vitamin A* used in anti-acne creams and gels — not as effective as *retinoic acid*

Retinoic acid:
A type of *vitamin A* used in anti-acne creams and gels and with skin-*rejuvenation* properties

Retinoids:
Any medicine or chemical related to *vitamin A*

Retinol:
A type of *vitamin A* used in anti-acne creams and gels — not as effective as *retinoic acid*

Retinyl palmitate:
A type of *vitamin A* used in non-prescription creams and gels

RF:
Radiofrequency

Roaccutane:
Brand name (used in the UK) of *isotretinoin*

Rosacea:
A skin disease, usually of the face, with skin redness and acne-like bumps

Rutinosides:
A particular chemical class of *antioxidant* derived from plants

Salicylic acid:
A common ingredient in creams, gels and lotions that reduces abnormal scale build-up in the skin and can also reduce redness in spots

Sculptra:
A treatment in which polymerised *lactic acid* is injected as a suspension to stimulate new skin *collagen* – used for *atrophic* sunken scar treatments

Sebaceous glands:
Glands under the skin, attached to hair follicles, that produce *sebum* – stimulated by *androgen hormones*

Sebaceous oil:
Sebum

Sebaceous oil ducts:
The tubes through which oil passes from the *sebaceous glands* to the surface of the skin. During acne development, these tubes sometimes become blocked and a blackhead or whitehead forms

Sebum:
The oily substance produced by sebaceous glands

Skin barrier:
A thin membrane of the outer skin that regulates water loss, skin moisture levels and prevents environmental toxins from entering the skin

SPF (sun protection factor):
The measure of how effectively a sunscreen prevents skin burning from sunlight, the higher the SPF – theoretically – the more protective. Our advice: a sunscreen with the maximum of SPF 50 is necessary on only *very* sunny days. SPF 15 – 20 is adequate on most UK days

Spironolactone:
A medicine mainly used as a *diuretic*, but also effective for reducing *androgen* effects in acne and unwanted body and face hair growth in women

Subcision:
A procedure in which a microscopic needle is used to sever the fibrous strands 'tethering' a sunken scar to the underlying tissues

Synergistic:
Having an enhanced effect in combination. Two or more ingredients are said to be synergistic if their combined effect is greater than the sum of their individual effects: so, if the effect of each alone was 2, their combined effect (2+2) might be 5

Tazarotene:
A very powerful *retinoid* gel or cream used for acne and *rejuvenation* of the skin

Telangiectasia:
Thread veins or visible smaller blood vessels

Teratogenic:
Potentially harmful to the developing *foetus*

Tetracyclines:
A group of *antibiotics* often used for treating acne

Tetralysal (*or* lymecycline):
An effective *antibiotic* used for acne

Thromboembolic disease:
Deep vein thrombosis

Tocopherol:
A form of *vitamin E* – a very effective *antioxidant*, both orally and as an ingredient in creams and gels

Topical:
(When describing medicine) anything that is applied directly to the

place that needs treatment; in **dermatology**, topical treatments are put straight on the skin rather than being taken by mouth

Tretinoin:
Another name for *retinoic acid*

Trimethoprim:
An *antibiotic* that can be used for treating acne

UVA (ultraviolet A):
The longest wavelengths of ultraviolet, which are responsible for skin ageing and skin darkening. Intense UVA may also increase the risk of skin cancer

Vascular:
Relating to blood vessels

Vitamin A:
A fat-soluble vitamin very important for the maintenance of normal skin formation

Vitamin B:
A group of water-soluble vitamins with many important functions. Two B vitamins used in skin creams are
    B3 (niacinamide) for acne and skin lightening,
    B5 (panthenol) for skin calming

Vitamin C:
An *antioxidant* vitamin present in fresh fruits and vegetables

Vitamin E:
An *antioxidant* vitamin derived from certain vegetables and oily foods

Willow bark:
A natural source of *salicylic acid*

Yasmin:

Brand name of an anti-acne **oral** contraceptive

Yaz:

Another brand name for **Yasmin**

Zinc:

A supplement or cream ingredient that is important for normal skin functions and cell production

INDEX

W

whiteheads 105
witch hazel 45, 48, 75

Z

zinc 28, 48, 49, 87, 118
zinc PCA 48, 49